The Achilles' Heel of the Biomedical Paradigm

James McCumiskey

Paperback edition first published in Great Britain
in 2021 by James McCumiskey.

eBook edition first published in Great Britain
in 2021 by James McCumiskey.

ISBN: 9798750626779

James McCumiskey

To my wonderful wife,

Donna McCumiskey

Contents

Introduction

At the time of writing, we are over 18 months into the Corona Crisis. There are many new words and phrases describing our current predicament such as COVID, lockdown, social distancing, self-isolate, close contact, shielding, curfew, compulsory mask wearing, bubbles, asymptomatic carrier, shedding, pingdemic, long-COVID etc. New variants of the SARS-CoV-2 virus are appearing, which are more virulent than previous versions.

As a consequence of the lockdowns people said 'stay safe' or 'be safe' at the end of a conversation meaning that you should avoid meeting or being in contact with other people so as not to become infected. There was a palpable feeling of fear during the first lockdown because we were living in 'troubling or unprecedented times'. The conventional wisdom is that lockdowns are ethically correct because they prevent many unnecessary deaths from COVID-19. Government and the media have conditioned us to disparage anyone who does not obey the COVID-19 regulations as being criminally negligent and immoral. Governments have deprived us of our liberties to keep us safe and the vast majority of us are grateful.

I am an accountant. I have no formal medical training whatsoever. Sixteen years ago, I came across the work of Dr Stefan Lanka PhD. He made what I then believed was an astounding and outlandish claim that there is no scientific evidence supporting the existence of pathogenic viruses. He then wrote, and he always writes, that we should not accept his word but investigate for ourselves. I have investigated and confirmed his claim; viruses do not exist.

When one discusses the idea that the SARS-CoV-2 virus does not exist, most people instinctively become emotional and cannot rationally deal with the issue.

What about all the people who died?

I tested positive. Surely, I must have had COVID?

I had COVID symptoms and I tested positive. How dare you say that the virus does not exist!

I lost my sense of smell and taste and tested positive. I had COVID.

What do you know? You are neither a doctor nor a virologist.

I had shortness of breath and a fever and no energy; I could not move for a few weeks. I tested positive. I definitely had COVID. What makes you think I did not?

I was infected, then my husband. His parents were very ill and had to be hospitalised. We all tested positive for COVID. We must all have had COVID. We must have infected each other; the virus must have spread from one person to another and infected the entire family.

Take a deep breath. Take a few long deep breaths. Calm down. I do not deny that you or your family members or friends got ill or unfortunately, some may even have died, and that their death-certificate states that the cause of death was COVID. I do not deny that many people tested positive for SARS-CoV-2. I do not deny reality; I do not deny what happened. What I emphatically deny is that a virus called SARS-CoV-2 caused the deaths and illnesses.

Please leave emotion to one side and the fact that you may currently believe that the SARS-CoV-2 virus exists and that it infected you or a loved one. This book is for those who want to examine the science behind the belief in the existence of viruses objectively, rationally and unemotionally.

The Achilles' Heel

In Greek mythology Achilles was a hero of the Trojan War and the central character of Homer's Iliad. Achilles died from a heel wound caused by an arrow.

His bizarre death inspired a number of legends as to how he was fatally wounded in such an odd way. According to one legend, his mother dipped the infant Achilles into a river, holding onto him by his heel, and he became invulnerable where the waters touched him; that is, everywhere but the areas on his heel covered by her thumb and forefinger. Another legend has it that his mother rubbed his body with ambrosia and then held him over a fire every night. She held him by his heel, which is why that part of his body was vulnerable.

These legends have caused the expression 'an Achilles' heel' to become a cliché, used to describe an area of weakness or an especially vulnerable spot. An Achilles' heel is a weakness in spite of overall strength, which can lead to downfall. For example, in popular culture, Superman only looses his super-human strength against kryptonite, which is his great weakness.

The Biomedical Paradigm

The word paradigm means a set of assumptions, concepts, values and practices, which constitute a way of viewing reality. Modern medicine is also called allopathy or allopathic medicine. Allopathic medicine is the treatment of disease by conventional means, by using drugs, surgery, radiotherapy etc to counteract the symptoms. The Biomedical Paradigm is the belief system underpinning allopathic medicine. According to these beliefs, germs, faulty genes and carcinogens cause disease.

The Germ Theory of Disease

The Germ Theory of Disease is the central belief of the Biomedical Paradigm. The Germ Theory of Disease states that germs cause disease that viruses cause viral diseases and bacteria cause bacterial diseases. Accordingly, the HIV-virus causes AIDS and the respective viruses cause mumps, measles, rubella and chickenpox.

Our belief in the Germ Theory of Disease compels us to vaccinate our children. Our belief in the existence of pathogenic viruses has permitted belief in a deadly new virus called SARS-CoV-2, which causes the disease COVID-19 and has necessitated the worldwide lockdowns.

The Achilles' Heel of the Biomedical Paradigm

Allopathic medicine and its underlying belief system—the Biomedical Paradigm—is seemingly impregnable and invincible in its control over us mere mortals, especially since the onset of COVID-19.

However, the Achilles' Heel of the Biomedical Paradigm is that viruses; pathogenic viruses; disease-inducing viruses; viruses that allegedly cause diseases such as COVID-19, AIDS, mumps, measles, rubella, polio, swine-flu and bird-flu do not exist!

The Biomedical Paradigm

The Biomedical Paradigm is the series of beliefs underpinning medicine and biology. The central belief of the Biomedical Paradigm is the Germ Theory of Disease; Germs cause disease, bacteria cause bacterial infections and viruses cause viral infections. The next most important belief is vaccination because it prevents infectious diseases. However, these beliefs are not rooted in scientific reality but rather in scientific fraud and misconceptions.

Those who fail to learn from history are doomed to repeat it.

Winston Churchill (British statesman, 1874–1965)

I assured the Emperor that all my ambition was to arrive at the knowledge of the causes of putrid and contagious diseases.

The greatest derangement of the mind is to believe in something because one wishes it to be so.

The microbe is nothing; the terrain is everything.

Louis Pasteur (French chemist and microbiologist, 1822–1895)

The most serious disorders may be provoked by the injection of living organisms into the blood.

Disease is born of us and in us.

Antoine Béchamp (French scientist and doctor, 1816–1908)

An error can never become true however many times you repeat it. The truth can never be wrong, even if no one ever hears about it.

Mahatma Gandhi (Indian statesman, 1869–1947)

Chapter 1

The Germ Theory of Disease

The Corona Crisis has brought the issue of viruses to the fore. We were all educated to believe that viruses exist and that vaccinations eliminated infectious diseases. The vast majority of us have had our children vaccinated because we implicitly believe in the existence of pathogenic viruses.

Likewise, all our doctors, nurses, virologists, microbiologists and other medics believed in the existence of viruses before they received their formal professional training. Their medical training confirmed and reinforced their pre-existing belief in the Germ Theory of Disease.

We need to understand how the Germ Theory of Disease came to be accepted as a scientific fact, and why it is false. Our belief in the existence of viruses comes from our belief in the Germ Theory of Disease.

The Miasma Theory of Disease

Prior to the Germ Theory of Disease, the predominant theory of infectious disease was miasmas or bad air. Accordingly, one believed that noxious miasmas, which originated from a foreign country or a remote place, caused cholera and the Black Plague. Interestingly, the word malaria comes from the Italian *'mal aria'* or bad air. Thus, the received wisdom was that 'bad air' transmits infectious diseases.

In the late 18th century, 'contagionists' challenged the miasma / bad-air theory. They claimed that disease was spread by human contact.

A case in point of the contrasting viewpoints between contagionists and anti-contagionists is the yellow fever epidemic that occurred in Philadelphia in 1793. It killed up to 5,000 people, or about 10% of the population. Many of the city's residents, including George Washington, fled the city during the outbreak. Benjamin Rush, a doctor and co-signatory of the US Declaration of Independence, stayed put and helped his fellow citizens. Rush angered his fellow doctors by arguing that yellow fever was not caused by contagion (human-human transmission), but from poisoning by putrid matter. He was correct. Yellow fever is not an infectious disease, rather is a water-borne disease, which for example can be caused by dead rotting animals in the water.

The Greek word *miasma* means pollution. The sanitation reformers in the mid-1800s in London, England, adapted the miasma viewpoint of the origin of 'infectious' disease from that of bad air to bad drinking water and non-existent sanitation / waste disposal systems. They were concerned to improve sanitation as a means of controlling disease and improving the quality of life.

There were numerous cholera epidemics prior to this time. Once these sanitary reforms were introduced, cholera and other allegedly infectious diseases were eliminated and death rates declined dramatically.

The belief in the miasma theory of disease was positively transformed from that of bad air to dirty water and bad sanitation causing 'infectious' disease. However, the belief persisted that the air carried infectious disease, this time by germs in the air, rather than by the air itself.

Origin of the Germ Theory of Disease

In 1683, a Dutch naturalist and lens maker, Anton van Leeuwenhoek, made the first recorded observations of microorganisms. In 1762, Marcus Antonius Plenciz, a Viennese physician, first published a germ theory of infectious diseases, which speculated that a specific microorganism caused a particular disease, and that they might be conveyed by air (Pearson, page 12).

Louis Pasteur is credited with the invention of the Germ Theory of Disease in the late 1870s. However, the Germ Theory of Disease was discussed in medical and scientific circles prior to the official recognition of Louis Pasteur's claim. For example, Florence Nightingale (the famous English nurse and social reformer) attacked the idea of contagion in 1860 (Pearson, page 12).

The Germ Theory of Disease developed from the Germ Theory of Fermentation as advanced by Louis Pasteur. At this time, there was a widely accepted analogy between fermentation and disease. Even today, this is not too hard to imagine. Fermentation and disease are similar processes. Disease can be regarded is a process of putrefaction—a process of breaking down the host organism. This meant that if one understood the cause of fermentation one would understand the causes of disease.

Fermentation means the conversion of sugar to alcohol using yeast. A more accurate definition would be the chemical conversion of carbohydrates into alcohols or acids. Fermentation is the process used to produce wine, beer and vinegar, among other things.

In May 1854, Professor Antoine Béchamp investigated why cane sugar was transformed at room temperature into grape sugar when dissolved in water. The idea that prevailed at the time was that this transformation occurred spontaneously at room temperature. Grape sugar is a solution of equal parts of glucose and fructose. The technical term for this change is inversion. Thus, the grape sugar was also known as invert sugar (Pearson, page 15).

Béchamp dissolved pure sugar cane in a glass bottle containing some air, but which was otherwise air-tight. As a control experiment, he had several other glass bottles containing the same solution but with a chemical added. The capped bottles were placed alongside each other in the laboratory. In the bottle without any added chemicals, moulds appeared within 30 days and inversion of the sugar then developed rapidly. The added chemicals prevented the moulds and the inversion of sugar in the other bottles. He published these observations in the Report of the French Academy of Science in February 1855 (Pearson, page 15).

He started a second set of experiments in June 1856 in order to determine the origin of the moulds. In two bottles, he had some air in contact with the solution. In nine other bottles, there was no air. The results were conclusive. In the nine bottles without air, no moulds were formed and no inversion of the sugar occurred. In the two bottles with air, he observed again that inversion occurred (Pearson, page 16).

These experiments proved beyond doubt that moulds and inversion of the sugar cane did not occur spontaneously. Rather it must have been because of something in the air. The moulds were living organisms and the cane sugar became inverted in proportion to the development of the moulds.

In 1856, it was generally accepted that fermentation could only occur with the presence of nitrogen. However, Béchamp's solutions contained pure water and cane sugar. They did not contain nitrogen or any other minerals. Therefore, Béchamp had proved that the mould grew because it had absorbed nitrogen from the air. It would have been astonishing news at the time that microbes absorbed nitrogen from the air, which then developed into moulds, fermented and caused the inversion or transformation of the sugar.

Béchamp explained the phenomenon of fermentation as being due to the nutrition of living organisms; a process of absorption, assimilation and excretion. The airborne germs 'planted' themselves in the sugared solution, absorbed nitrogen from the air and developed fungi or moulds.

Béchamp referred to the mould as the insoluble ferment because it did not dissolve in water. The soluble ferment dissolved into the water and caused the inversion or transformation of the solution. Thus, fermentation is an effect accompanying the growth of the mould.

The dates mentioned above for Professor Béchamp's experiments are relevant because in 1860 Louis Pasteur engaged upon a theatrical series of experiments to demonstrate what Béchamp had already proven a few years earlier. He gave public notice of his proposed experiment. He prepared 73 bottles of unfermented liquid, which he exposed to the air in different places at various altitudes. He opened the bottles and then sealed them to capture the air at those locations. He opened the last 20 bottles in a spectacular location, a glacier called Mer de Glace above Chamonix. The results were as Béchamp had proved several years earlier (Pearson, page 20).

Pasteur had one interesting addition to this experiment. He borrowed the idea of a 'swan-neck' bottle flask from a colleague. This specially made flask would only allow germ-free and dust-free air into the liquid solution, the airborne germs settling in the horizontal part of the swan-neck at the top of the flask. No fermentation took place in the solution in the swan-neck flask, proving that one needed airborne germs for fermentation to occur (Pearson, page 20).

In 1860, with his well-publicised 'high Alps' experiment, Pasteur stole credit for Béchamp's discovery that germs in the air caused fermentation. In 1861, at the Sorbonne in Paris, he had the audacity, in the presence of Béchamp himself, to take credit for what Béchamp had discovered a few years earlier. "Béchamp asked him to admit knowledge of Béchamp's 1857 work, but did not charge him with plagiarism, and Pasteur evaded the question ... however, Béchamp was too much of a gentleman to make any unpleasant charges" (Pearson, page 21).

Pasteur erroneously concluded that each kind of fermentation (milk, beer or wine) had a specific germ (Pearson, page 23). In this context, it is not surprising that Pasteur believed that if airborne germs were the cause of fermentation that they had to be the cause of disease. The Germ Theory of Disease developed from this hypothesis.

In 1863, Pasteur was elected to the Academy of Science. Soon afterwards, he had an audience with the French Emperor. Pasteur wrote in a letter the next day, "I assured the Emperor that all my ambition was to arrive at the knowledge of the causes of putrid and contagious diseases" (Hume, page 165).

Béchamp's Microzymas

Béchamp discovered that when he added chemically pure calcium carbonate (CaCO3) to his sugared solutions, no inversion occurred, but when ordinary chalk chipped off from a rock was used, inversion always occurred (Pearson, page 26).

The chalk (comprised of calcium carbonate) found in Nature also contained what he called "little bodies" or "microzymas". The name microzymas comes from the Greek for 'small' and 'ferment'. They were smaller than anything he had seen in the moulds before. Because they moved and caused fermentation, he regarded them as living organisms. The block of limestone, from which he obtained the chalk, was very old. These microzymas had remained dormant in the limestone for thousands if not millions of years, and were the survivors of living beings from long ago.

Béchamp isolated the microzymas and determined their composition from carbon, hydrogen etc. If the ferments found in ordinary chalk were living beings, it had to be possible to kill them. He heated the chalk together with some water to 300 degrees centigrade and found that the microzymas were killed off and no fermentation took place (Hume, page 174).

Béchamp had already proved that creosote prevented external airborne organisms from entering the medium. However, when he added creosote in with the ordinary chalk, inversion still occurred. This was an unexpected result. The microzymas appeared in chalk found in Nature but were not present in chemically pure calcium carbonate (Hume, page 173).

In early 1868, Professor Béchamp and his colleague Professor Estor tested their theories on the origin of microzymas. They obtained the body of a dead kitten and buried it in pure carbonate of lime, which was treated to exclude airborne germs. They placed this entombed dead kitten in a glass jar. They covered the top of the jar with several sheets of paper, which were arranged to allow air but to prevent dust or other airborne germs from entering. The jar was left on a shelf in the laboratory for seven years until the end of 1874. When they opened it, they found that the kitten's body had been almost entirely consumed with the exception of some small fragments of bones. There was no smell and the carbonate of lime was not discoloured (Pearson, page 28).

They observed no microzymas above the kitten's body, but there were thousands below it. Béchamp thought there might have been airborne germs in the kitten's fur, lungs, or intestines. He repeated the same experiment using the carcass of a kitten in one case, the liver in another and the heart, lungs and kidneys in a third. These experiments started in 1875 and ended seven years later in 1882.

Again, with the exclusion of airborne germs, Béchamp and Estor discovered seven years later that microzymas were also present.

These series of experiments proved that microzymas are the living remnants of plant and animal life (Hume, pages 203-204).

Béchamp was the first scientist to explain the fermentative power of airborne germs. He also demonstrated how fermentation could occur without the presence of airborne germs (Hume, page 201).

Béchamp and Bacteria

Professor Béchamp and Professor Estor found bacteria present in their experiments. Because they had taken care to exclude airborne germs, they deduced that bacteria develop from microzymas. Bacteria are in fact a scavenging form of these microzymas; developed when tissue needs to be repaired or broken up. The bacteria were created from the microzymas, which in turn came from the decomposing body of the dead kitten (Pearson, page 29).

In the 1860s, scientists discovered bacteria in the tissue and blood of patients with typhoid fever, gangrene and anthrax. Scientists interpreted the presence of bacteria as being the cause of these diseases, and that the bacteria had invaded the organism from outside, carried by the air. However, the interpretation of Béchamp and Estor was that the cells in the body itself had changed and produced bacteria in response to the conditions of the host organism (Pearson, page 29).

Béchamp's microzymas, including specific bacteria, could take on a number of forms during the host's life cycle and these forms depended primarily on the chemistry of their environment, on the biological terrain, or on the condition of the host.[1]

Bacteria in man or animal do not cause disease. They have the same function as those found in the soil, in sewage or elsewhere in Nature. They exist in order to rebuild dead or diseased tissues or eliminate body waste. Bacteria do not and cannot attack healthy tissue (Pearson, page 30).

Béchamp also argued strenuously against vaccines, asserting: "The most serious disorders may be provoked by the injection of living organisms into the blood."[2]

Béchamp was the first scientist to discover that airborne germs cause fermentation. Pasteur wrongly deduced that airborne germs cause all diseases. Béchamp had proven that small germs (microzymas) contained in ordinary chalk could cause fermentation when airborne germs were excluded. He also discovered that microzymas were obtained from the decomposition of a dead animal, excluding airborne germs, and that bacteria developed from these microzymas. He had a much more nuanced version of germs than Pasteur had, and rejected the simplistic notion that airborne germs cause disease.

---

1 Biological Terrain vs The Germ Theory, hosted by http://thehealthadvantage.com. Retrieved March 2021.
2 Biological Terrain vs The Germ Theory, hosted by http://thehealthadvantage.com. Retrieved March 2021.

Claude Bernard and Pasteur

In 1878, Claude Bernard, a friend and scientific colleague of Pasteur, died. One of Bernard's colleagues instigated the publication of his laboratory notes which disputed Pasteur's purely airborne germ theory of fermentation. Claude Bernard had never challenged Pasteur's theory while alive. Pasteur was then 55-years-old, a French hero with a huge reputation and ego. Pasteur repeated Bernard's experiments and produced a devastating critique of Bernard in both tone and substance. Part of his critique was about the dangers of preconceived ideas, or of believing what you want to believe to be true. By contrast, Pasteur presented himself as a true scientist, working empirically with no preconceived theories (Geison, pages 18-20).

In fact, any analysis of Pasteur's own work shows that he conducted his own experiments according to his own preconceived ideas and rejected experiments that did not fit in with the result he had expected—the exact opposite of what a true scientist should do (Geison, page 16).

Because of the posthumous publication of Bernard's notes and the ensuing furore, and probably influenced by worries over being called a fraud and a plagiarist, Pasteur instructed his family to keep his laboratory notebooks private (Geison, pages 19-20).

Pasteur died 18 years later in 1895. On his deathbed, his diatribe against Claude Bernard must have been on his mind. He is alleged to have said "Bernard is right: the microbe is nothing: the terrain is everything."[3] In other words, microbes do not cause disease; they are merely present during disease. However, it was too late. The Germ Theory of Disease, which he invented and promulgated, was now in the ascendancy.

Challenging the Germ Theory of Disease

The German chemist and hygienist Max von Pettenkofer (1818-1901) obtained a cholera culture from the Koch Institute without revealing his true intention. On 7 October 1892, the 74 year old drank a millilitre of these cholera bacilli. He did not get sick nor did he get cholera. His assistant repeated the same experiment on 17 October 1892. He got slightly sick but recovered rapidly. He too did not get cholera (Widmer, page 44).

Cholera bacilli do not cause cholera; they are present when the patient is suffering from cholera. Max Von Pettenkofer's bold, brave and effective experiment did not convince his contemporaries because of the strength of their belief in the Germ Theory of Disease. Their counter explanation would have been that although germs cause disease, the 74-year-old Max Von Pettenkofer must have had a strong immune system.

The Germ Theory of Disease was hotly debated at the time, but because of their conviction that disease was caused by

3 Pasteur's deathbed saying is quoted in many articles on the internet. It could be a case of projection. It could be simply ascribed to him, as something he might well have said, if he had recanted on his deathbed.

external factors and not by internal factors, the medical and scientific community came to accept it as scientific truth.

It was a lost chapter in the history of biology and medicine that the original scientific work of Professors Béchamp and Estor was discarded in favour of Louis Pasteur.

Cellular Pathology

Cellular Theory assumes that the basic structural unit of all organisms is the cell: All life (humans, animals and plants) develops from a cell. Cellular Theory is the basis for molecular genetics, where genes are the building blocks of life. Cellular Theory is also the basis for cancer theories, radiation and chemotherapy (Lanka, 2015:2).

Rudolf Virchow obtained his ideas on Cellular Theory from the atomic theory of the Greek philosophers Democritus and Epicurus. He claimed analogous to the atomic theory that all life originates from a cell. The cell was the smallest indivisible unit of life, which would also cause diseases by creating toxins; this theory is called Cellular Pathology (Lanka, 2020:3).

One cannot understate the importance of Cellular Pathology in medicine and biology today.

In 1855, Robert Remak discovered the relationship between diseases and the embryonic germ layers. Three years later, in 1858, Virchow suppressed this knowledge and invented his theory of Cellular Pathology, which is currently accepted as a scientific fact. Dr Stefan Lanka calls this act by Virchow a "brutal plagiarism" because of all the hardship and suffering it has subsequently caused (Lanka, 2015:2).

Cellular Pathology assumes that all diseases originate in cells. According to this theory, the cell produces a pathogen, which spreads to other cells in the body and then from one person to another causing contagion (Lanka, 2015:2).

However, contrary to current scientific opinion, life does not develop from cells rather from the embryonic germ layers. The germ layers are formed first and then rudimentary parts of the organs. Then, the cells are formed; they divide and differentiate themselves. The interaction of these germ layers creates all living beings (humans, animals and plants) and is called embryology. Three germ layers are created in the first fifteen days of the life of a new embryo. These three germ layers are the endoderm or inner germ layer, the mesoderm or middle germ layer, and the ectoderm or outer germ layer. The three germ layers can be broadly classified as serving the four basic principles of life: digestion, protection, movement and contact (Lanka, 2015:2).

Dr Ryke Geerd Hamer MD (1935-2017) re-discovered the importance of the embryonic germ layers in the early 1980s and used them to classify all diseases.[4] Dr Hamer also realised that microbes work symbiotically and are used to optimise healing. There is no such thing as bad bacteria or good bacteria. All bacteria are good. The microbes that

4 The Third Biological Law: The Ontogenetic System of the Biological Programmes.

do exist such as fungi, bacteria and mycobacteria always work for our benefit.[5]

Dr Ryke Geerd Hamer's body of work is known by different names, originally New Medicine, then German New Medicine, and finally before he died, he renamed it *Germanische Heilkunde* or the German Art of Healing. The cornerstone of his work are the Five Biological Laws, which explains the course of every disease known to man; why we get the cancer or disease and the progression to death or full recovery. The strength of the medical profession's belief in the Germ Theory of Disease and Cellular Pathology has to date prevented them from verifying and then accepting the Five Biological Laws.

The Central Beliefs of Medicine and Biology

The Germ Theory of Disease is the central belief of medicine and biology. Cellular Pathology is a very closely associated belief, whereby the cell is the building block of life and disease originates in the cells.

The Germ Theory of Disease and Cellular Pathology are the core beliefs of medicine and biology. Pasteur established the Germ Theory of Disease by plagiarising the work of Béchamp. However, his Germ Theory of Disease did accord with the long held idea of miasmas or bad air causing infectious disease. Likewise, Virchow suppressed the importance of the embryonic germ layers in the classification of disease and came up with Cellular Pathology,

5 The Fourth Biological Law: The Ontogenetic System of Microbes.

which also did accord with long-held beliefs about the cell being the basic unit of life.

The Germ Theory of Disease and Cellular Pathology are false. The belief in these scientific theories has led medicine and biology to a dead-end, to virus mania and the Corona Crisis. Our belief in these theories has resulted in our firm conviction that pathogenic viruses exist.

According to the Cellular Pathology theory, viruses are created in a cell, spread from one cell to another, thereby infecting the whole body and are transmissible from one human to another. Thus, the SARS-CoV-2 virus causes a range of diseases called COVID-19 and spreads from one human to another causing the current pandemic.

Our belief in the Existence of Viruses

There was a worldwide influenza pandemic in 1889-90. "There seems to be general agreement that this pandemic had most of the characteristics of the greater one in 1918 except for its lower fatality". Dr Richard Pfeiffer, a German physician and bacteriologist, discovered a bacterium, *Haemophilus influenza,* which was subsequently called Pfeiffer's bacillus, which he believed was the cause of influenza, "because according to him, it was present in all cases and not present in normal individuals unless they had recently recovered from influenza ..... Pfeiffer's view were widely accepted, and it is safe to say that the majority of medical people at the time believed that he had discovered the cause of influenza" (Shope, 1958).

"Much work was expended during the 1918 pandemic in an effort to determine the causative agent of the outbreak.

Prior to the 1918 studies *Haemophilus influenza* had been generally regarded as the agent responsible for influenza....With the failure to gain clear-cut evidence that *Haemophilus influenza* was the cause of the 1918 pandemic, the view was rather widely held and was frequently expressed that a virus was probably the etiological basis for the disease" (Shope, 1958).

Thus, the scientists and doctors believed that a virus had to be the cause of the 1918 influenza pandemic. Likewise, when the doctors could not discover bacteria when a patient presented with mumps, measles, rubella or polio, they believed that a virus must be the causative agent. Their belief in the existence of viruses was because of their belief in the Germ Theory of Disease. If bacteria could not be observed when the patient was ill, then they believed that a virus had to be the causative agent.

Our belief in the existence of pathogenic viruses predated our ability to detect them. All alleged pathogenic viruses range in size from 20nm to 200nm in diameter. A nanometere is one billionth of a metre.

In contrast, bacteria range in size from 500nm to 2,000nm. Thus, bacteria are an order of magnitude bigger than all alleged pathogenic viruses. Bacteria exist; they have been isolated, their dimensions measured, photographed and biochemically characterised.

The electron microscope became available for scientific use in 1938. Electron microscopes were invented because light microscopes are limited by the physics of light to a resolution of 200nm. An electron microscope uses electrons instead of light for the imaging of objects. Electron microscopes currently have a resolution of 0.2nm[6].

If pathogenic viruses existed, it would be possible to view them using an electron microscope and photograph them. Dr Lanka has repeatedly stated in his writings that nobody has ever observed a virus using an electron microscope and photographed it. It does not matter whether the sample is from a human, animal or plant or in any liquids from them such as blood, semen, saliva etc, nobody has ever observed or photographed a virus.[7]

Even if one questions what Dr Lanka says and still believes that a virus must be present in a blood sample, tissue sample or saliva sample, it should be possible to isolate it. By the word 'isolate' we mean to separate the virus from all other component parts in the sample. Nobody has ever isolated any alleged pathogenic virus.[8]

The reason why it has not been possible neither to observe, photograph nor to isolate any alleged pathogenic virus is that they are fictitious theoretical constructs with no basis in biological reality.

---

6 Resolution of an Electron Microscope - The Physics Factbook http://hypertextbook.com/facts/2000/IlyaSherman.shtml Retrieved September 2021.

7 This is elaborated in Chapter 5: Viruses Cannot Exist.

8 This is elaborated in Chapter 6: No Record Exists.

Chapter 2

Vaccination

The underlying belief of vaccination is to use the body's immune system to protect it from infectious diseases. The idea is to cause a mild form of the disease because of a mistaken belief in 'immunity'. If you get the disease once, even a weakened form of it, you are believed to be immune for life.

The practice of 'vaccination' was originally called 'inoculation', which came about because of smallpox.

Inoculation

Smallpox is, according to received wisdom, a highly contagious disease unique to humans. The main symptoms are persistent skin scarring resulting in very visible pockmarks all over the body. Many survivors are left blind in one or both eyes. Smallpox was responsible for millions of deaths in the 20th century alone.

The first attempts at inoculation were recorded in China a thousand years ago. Inoculation involved purposely infecting a person with a mild form of smallpox. Inoculation was from person to person. The first form of inoculation was that healthy people would inhale a powder made from the crusts of smallpox scabs in order to protect themselves. Laterally, this procedure involved transferring the smallpox postule or pus from a person suffering from a mild form of smallpox onto a scratch between the thumb and forefinger of a healthy person. Inoculation reached Europe in the 1700s, where it was also called variolation, after the Latin name for smallpox—variola.[9]

Lady Mary Wortley-Montagu lost a brother to smallpox and her face was scared by it. Thus, she had a strong motive to prevent the disease. While in Constantinople, when her husband was the British Ambassador to the Ottoman Empire, she witnessed the widespread practice of inoculation and was so greatly impressed that she had her son inoculated in 1718. On her return to England, Lady Montagu campaigned for the introduction of this prophylactic or preventative procedure (Widmer, page 18).

Thousands more people died in London from this procedure than from smallpox itself. By 1727, there were descriptions of smallpox outbreaks because of inoculation (Widmer, page 19). Nevertheless, despite all the evidence to the contrary, there was this mistaken belief in immunity fortified by the doctors and others carrying out this procedure, but also as a generally accepted belief by the public. The practice of inoculation (from person to person) continued until the discovery of 'vaccination' by Edward Jenner in the late 1700s.

Vaccination

Edward Jenner (1749–1823) is considered to be the father of vaccination. Jenner observed that dairy farmers did not get smallpox. He hypothesised that prior infection with cowpox—a mild illness spread from cattle—might be responsible for the perceived immunity against smallpox.

9 https://www.etymonline.com/ Retrieved February 2021.

He made a series of experiments where he tested his hypothesis. He injected the cowpox pus from cows directly into the patient's vein. Jenner called his discovery *vaccination*, the word deriving from *vacca,* the Latin for cow.

In 1790, Jenner vaccinated his 10-month-old son in this fashion. His son was thereafter mentally handicapped and died at age 21. Jenner's firm belief in vaccination blinded him against the terrible consequences. At the end of his life, he expressed doubts about what he had done, but the practice of vaccination was a much too profitable a business for his colleagues (Widmer, page 20).

Symptoms such as fever, skin rash, diarrhoea and vomiting were initially understood by people to be a sign that the vaccine was damaging them. Edward Jenner reinterpreted the symptoms and claimed they were a sign that the vaccine had 'taken' and was working successfully. Eventually people accepted this idea as 'proof' that a vaccine was effective (Stoll, page 71).

Dr Archie Kalokerinos, an Australian doctor and ardent vaccine critic, states that the death rate and the severe injuries from Jenner's vaccinations would be enormous if carried out today. There is a huge body of evidence to support the reality that vaccination significantly increased the death rate (Sinclair, foreword)

The Belief in Immunity

The whole theory of vaccinations is rooted in the belief that a non-fatal attack of a disease confers immunity.

This theory arose for two reasons. Firstly, medicine considered disease to be an entity, a definite thing in itself, which has to be fought. Secondly, medicine obtained the idea of immunity from the observed facts over many thousands of years that most children only get diseases such as measles, mumps, rubella or chicken pox once and that some kind of protection has been given them to prevent any further occurrences. This belief in immunity from a naturally occurring disease (such as measles) occurring more than once was then transferred over to a belief in vaccinations. They believed that the perceived immunity, which occurs from ordinary diseases, could be artificially replicated by vaccination.

Thus, the current belief is that by injecting a child with a mild form of the 'virus', the immune system is stimulated. It produces antibodies against this weakened or, in technical terms, attenuated form of the virus. These antibodies are present so that in the future, when the child's immune system comes across the real measles, mumps and rubella viruses, for example, it can immediately fight them off providing immunity.

Over thousands of years, human experience would indicate that the child having had measles, mumps and rubella is most unlikely to have them again. However, doctors, if they are honest, will admit that they have come across kids who have had measles two or three times whether vaccinated or not.

Vaccines are Ineffective

A vaccine introduces a weakened or inactive version of the infection into the body. Once vaccinated you should be immune to infection, which means that if you encounter the pathogen (bacteria or virus) your body has acquired the ability to fight off the infection before the disease takes hold.

Taking measles as an example, the measles vaccine is called an antigen, which allegedly stimulates the immune system to produce antibodies against the weakened or dead measles 'virus' contained in the vaccine. The supposed advantage of vaccination is that your immune system remembers the measles virus and can quickly create antibodies in the future to destroy a real live dangerous measles virus. Thus, you are protected from the real measles virus.

The proof presented by the virologists that the measles vaccine works is:

1. Most children in the developed world do not get measles because they have been vaccinated; and

2. Antibodies can be measured, which prove that the measles vaccine has been effective.

However, there are convincing explanations, which counter the virologists belief in the effectiveness of the measles vaccine, or indeed any other vaccine.

Antibodies

I found the word antibody to be something of a mystery. How could some small substance be against or anti the body? The scientists believe that an antibody is a "substance developed in blood as an antitoxin". Antibody comes from the German 'Antikörper', which is condensed from 'anti-toxischer Körper' or anti-toxic body.[10] Thus, the scientists believe that an anti-body is created in response to a toxin and is therefore an 'anti-toxin body' or antibody; it protects the body against the toxin.

The idea of a toxin causing disease is a few thousand years old as is the idea of the person being prophylactically treated to produce an antidote against the toxin. The antibody is the modern day antidote to various 'infectious' diseases.

Antibodies are proteins in the blood. They are also called globulins. They are used for the sealing of cells and tissues in the cases of injury and growth. They do not constitute protection from disease. There are no specific antibodies against a specific disease. Globulins can be made to coalesce or bind with other proteins in laboratory tests and in this way can be manipulated arbitrarily. Their binding ability is regarded by the scientists as proof that the vaccine has worked. However, the ability of the globulins to bind is solely dependent on the conditions in the test-tube and can be arbitrarily manipulated by the scientists (Stoll, page 112).

Vaccines contain multiple toxins. The human body creates globulins to protect it from the toxic effects of the vaccine. The increase in the number of globulins after vaccination is nothing more than a reaction of the body to its poisoning. The globulin count also rises after other types of poisoning such as from lead, mercury or chemotherapy.

10 https://www.etymonline.com/ Retrieved March 2021.

The toxins in the vaccine tear holes in the tissue and consequently damage them. The body creates globulins to repair the damaged cells and tissue, in order to reseal them (Stoll, page 113).

The word antibody is misleading. Antibodies are simply globulins, which the body creates when it has been poisoned, whether by vaccines or by other toxins. Antibodies are created in order to repair the damage done to cells and tissues by toxins.

The increase in the antibody count, or more accurately the globulin count, is a sure sign that the vaccine has poisoned the body, which is the exact opposite of what the doctors and scientists claim.

The Decline of 'Infectious' Diseases

The myth that vaccines are effective arose primarily because of the real reduction in both mortality and incidence of so-called infectious diseases since the introduction of vaccination. The doctors and the media repeatedly tell us this, so much so, that we nearly all believe it to be an absolute truth.

The doctors themselves believe this and write in their textbooks and brochures that vaccination has been the most effective action in reducing death rates among children. However, the death rate from measles had been falling dramatically long before vaccinations were introduced, and simply continued its long-term decline after the introduction of vaccinations. The decline in the death rate from all of these diseases long preceded the introduction of vaccinations against them.

In the early 1800s, in London England, almost 50% of children died before the age of five. The reasons for these deaths were attributed to poor housing conditions, polluted drinking water, inadequate sewage disposal and malnutrition (Sinclair, page 13).

Edwin Chadwick, a London lawyer, suggested that if improvements were made in the quality of drinking water, and if effective waste disposal, sanitary reform and a clean-up of the environment were carried out, that most epidemic diseases would disappear. The Public Health Act was introduced in 1848 in the UK because of Chadwick's work (Sinclair, page 13).

Dr Snow MD is hailed as the first epidemiologist. He discovered that the source of cholera in London during an epidemic in 1854 was a particular water pump. The areas of London supplied by the relatively clean upper Thames had much less incidences of cholera than those sections of the city supplied with water from the lower Thames, which was fouled by human sewage. Sanitary reform eliminated cholera in London (Sinclair, page 14).

Max von Pettenkofer initiated a similar clean up in Munich providing clean drinking water to all houses and setting up effective waste disposal. As a consequence of this work, the death rate from typhoid declined from 72 per million population in 1880 to 14 per million in 1898 (Sinclair, page 13).

Since 1893, in Hamburg, there has been a general decrease in infant mortality (with noticeable increases during both world wars) from a peak of almost 30% of live births to almost zero today. The sand-filtration of the water from the river Elbe started in 1893; it is responsible for the general decline and elimination of diseases like cholera, typhus and smallpox in the city of Hamburg. The reduction in these diseases is caused by an improvement in the hygiene of the drinking water and that of the wastewater (Buchwald, page 161).

Clean water and good sanitation prevents water-borne diseases such as typhoid, cholera and yellow fever. However, how do we explain the reduction in mortality from other so-called infectious diseases?

From the beginning of time, hunger would have been an everyday occurrence for most people. It was only banished by the introduction of intensive farming, which ensured adequate production of food in the mid-1800s throughout Europe (McKeown, pages 59-65).

So-called infectious diseases such as measles, mumps and rubella against which we vaccinate our children are not to be feared in a well-nourished and well-loved child.

The medical-pharmaceutical complex take credit for the decline in infectious diseases because of the efficacy of vaccines. In reality, we should honour the campaigners for sanitary reform and clean drinking water and the civil engineers who designed and built these facilities.

All Vaccines are Toxic

If you examine the anti-vaccine web sites, they nearly all focus on the dangers of vaccinations and in particular, the 'combo-vaccines' (the 5-in-1 and 3-in-1 vaccines). They also focus on the toxic content of the vaccines and the ensuing toxic overload because of the quantity of shots given. They rarely question the need for vaccines.

The usual trick of the health authorities (if there is a sudden increase in disorders deaths or diseases caused by vaccination) is to blame a 'bad vaccine' or a bad 'batch' of a good vaccine, but otherwise there is no problem. After all, vaccination is one of the most effective tools of allopathic medicine: Everyone knows that it has saved millions of lives.

However, the truth is otherwise. All vaccines contain toxins and are therefore dangerous. The only good vaccine is one that is never used. The important point with regard to vaccination is that it is scientifically un-necessary and at the very least pointless and a waste of money to vaccinate against phantom viruses.

On Monday, 19 September 2011, I was astonished to read an article in the Irish Times entitled 'Warning of more cases of flu vaccine disorder' by Genevieve Carberry. I was surprised, because I did not think the Irish Times would publish an article critical of vaccines.

The article was about a new support group called SOUND (Sufferers Of Unique Narcolepsy Disorder) for parents whose children developed a chronic sleeping disorder called narcolepsy after receiving the swine flu vaccine Pandemrix. SOUND wants "to help parents to identify if their children are affected and to lobby the health authorities to support those already diagnosed".

Narcolepsy is a chronic sleep disorder, characterized by an excessive urge to sleep at inappropriate times, such as while at work. The term narcolepsy derives from the French word narcolepsie', which was created by combining the Greek 'narkē', "numbness" or "stupor", and 'lepsis', "attack" or "seizure".[11]

> "We believe there are a lot more children in this country who are suffering from this condition who have not being diagnosed and parents are struggling to figure out what's wrong with their children," said chairwoman Mary Fitzpatrick, whose 14-year-old son was diagnosed with the sleeping disorder having received the vaccine almost two years ago.
>
> :
>
> More than 900,000 doses of Pandremix were administered by GPs (General Practitioners) in Ireland during the pandemic. The Irish Government gave indemnity cover to drug-maker GlaxoSmithKline.
>
> The HSE (Health Service Executive) has said use of the vaccine is no longer recommended, and this year's seasonal flu vaccine does not contain Pandemrix.

There was a sinister follow-up article in the Irish Times on Monday October 3 2011 by Dr Muiris Houston MD about the swine-flu vaccine Pandremix. I reproduce the article because it vividly illustrates the point that the official narrative was that Pandremix was a 'bad vaccine'. His article depressed me. This is truly an age of universal deceit. Just a bad vaccine, but all the other vaccines are fine. Now

11 http://en.wikipedia.org/wiki/Narcolepsy

that this vaccine is withdrawn, the seasonal vaccination program should continue apace, with no concerns.

> **Concerns over swine flu vaccine should not deter us from getting seasonal shot**[12]
>
> **ANALYSIS:** There is no longer a need for controversial vaccine Pandemrix to be administered.
>
> UNOFFICIALLY, EXPERTS here acknowledge a probable link between the vaccine Pandemrix and a disease called narcolepsy.
>
> While the official line from the Health Service Executive is that it continues to investigate a possible link, it is not unreasonable to assume that Ireland will eventually follow the lead of Finland and Sweden where studies have shown a six- to 13-fold increase in cases of narcolepsy among those immunised with the swine flu vaccine.
>
> Unlike the annual seasonal influenza vaccine, which contains three strains of flu virus, Pandemrix was produced as a single flu strain vaccine in a bid to head off the potential impact of the swine flu (H1N1) pandemic virus in 2009 and 2010.

12 https://www.irishtimes.com/news/concerns-over-swine-flu-vaccine-should-not-deter-us-from-getting-seasonal-shot-1.612453 Retrieved February 2021.

It was one of two vaccines given to "at-risk" groups of patients in Ireland. GPs here administered some 900,000 doses of Pandemrix during the period.

Because a strain of the swine flu virus is included in this year's seasonal flu vaccine, there is no longer a need for Pandemrix to be administered. The HSE has asked doctors to return any supplies they may still have.

Nonetheless, it seems the one-off swine flu vaccine may have caused narcolepsy in a tiny minority of those who received the shot. A lobby group, Sound (Sufferers of Unique Narcolepsy Disorder), has been launched with the aim of helping parents identify if their children are affected and to seek support for those already diagnosed.

Narcolepsy is a debilitating neurological disorder that causes excessive daytime sleepiness, sometimes accompanied by muscle weakness. To date, the Irish Medicines Board has confirmed 16 cases of the disease in individuals vaccinated with Pandemrix.

It would be a pity if the concerns about Pandemrix were to impact negatively on the numbers availing of this year's seasonal flu vaccine. The immunisation season is now in full swing in GPs' surgeries. This year it will additionally target those aged over 50 as well as all pregnant women. Immunising expectant

> mothers has been national policy in other countries for some time and the indications are the three-strain flu vaccine, which is not a "live" vaccine, is very safe. It has been shown to reduce hospitalisation in pregnant women exposed to the flu.
>
> In people with chronic underlying disease, especially those over 65, complications from flu are common and hospitalisation rates high. Currently available influenza vaccines provide 70-90 per cent protection against influenza in people less than 65-years-old. And while efficacy in older people is lower, the vaccine lessens the severity of flu and the likelihood of death from it.
>
> The lessons of the MMR debacle are relevant. We are still seeing outbreaks of measles and mumps following the collapse of immunisation rates following the now discredited claims of a vaccine link with autism. The Pandemrix experience does not warrant a similar overreaction.

I was sorely tempted to respond directly to Dr Muiris Houston MD over this article but I did not. There was no point. I had exhausted my one-way correspondence with him over many years. He replied to me once, thanking me for my "interesting feedback", but never subsequently engaged with me, despite the countless emails I sent him and copied him about the fact that no one had ever isolated a virus.

Children who are not Vaccinated

All vaccines contain toxins and are therefore dangerous. There is no safe vaccine. The only safe vaccine is one that is never used.

Autism does not only occur because of one vaccine only such as the MMR vaccine but can occur from any vaccine or the cumulative effect of all vaccines. The way to prove the truth of this statement is to examine communities where the children are not vaccinated and observe the rate of autism.

One control group (the majority of the US population) fully vaccinate their children. Two different control groups, the Amish and the patients of a Chicago medical practice do not vaccinate their children.

The difference in autism rates between the vaccinated and the unvaccinated are staggering. Journalist Dan Olmstead examined the autism rate of the Amish in Lancaster County Pennsylvania in April 2005. Olmstead estimated that about 130 Amish should have autism, given the US national rate of autism. He found only four cases of autism. One child had been exposed to high levels of mercury from a power plant. The other three—including one child adopted from outside the Amish community—had received their vaccines.

Olmsted found a family MD in Lancaster County, Pennsylvania, who indicated that he had never seen an Amish person with autism (Olmstead, 2005).

Olmstead visited other Amish communities in the US. The Amish community around Middlefield, Ohio have an autism rate of 1 in 15,000, according to the medical director at a clinic for special needs children there. In contrast, the US national autism rate was then estimated at 1 in 166.

Homefirst Health Services in Chicago have two things in common with Amish children; they have never been vaccinated and they do not have autism. The Homefirst medical practice has six doctors in Chicago. "We have about 30,000 or 35,000 children that we've taken care of over the years, and I don't think we have a single case of autism in children delivered by us who never received vaccines," said Dr Mayer Eisenstein, Homefirst's medical director, who founded the practice in 1973 (Olmstead, 2005).

This is truly astonishing and is difficult for doctors to explain away. There is no autism in children who had never been vaccinated.

Let us extend the experiment further: Are there any cases of Sudden Infant Death Syndrome (SIDS), Shaken Baby Syndrome (SBS), attention deficit disorders, dyslexia in the unvaccinated groups? I am certain that the results would mirror that for autism.

Vaccination: A Business Based on Fear

Dr Gerhard Buchwald MD was a regular doctor who believed in the efficacy of vaccines. He was almost 40-years-old, when his eldest son, born in 1957, received a smallpox vaccination at the age of 18 months. Until then, his son had developed normally. Eight days after the smallpox vaccination, his son could no longer stand up in his cot. His son had post-vaccination encephalitis and Dr Buchwald had since then a "completely destroyed human being at home."[13]

Dr Buchwald has spent over 40 years researching the toxic effects of all vaccines. He documented these in his book: *Vaccination a Business based on Fear.* They all damage, some more than others do. The combination-vaccines are more dangerous than the single-dose vaccines, but they are all dangerous.

> ...The damage and the deaths caused by vaccinations are written off as "pure coincidence", as something which would have occurred anyway, even without vaccinations. Often damage is trivialised by claiming that vaccine damage occurs only very, very rarely, or the damage is covered up by naming as the cause the most unlikely syndromes, which can only be found in special literature. Most people do not know what form vaccine damage may take. For this reason, the...claims for compensation for vaccine damage registered with the welfare offices...are only the tip of an iceberg. Most of the damaged children disappear in institutions. The actual numbers is considerably higher. The bottom line is that this "public health measure" is BIG BUSINESS: A BUSINESS BASED ON FEAR (Buchwald, back cover).

---

13 Dr Buchwald's testimony before the Quebec College of Physicians Medical Board. http://www.whale.to. Retrieved April 2021.

Dr Buchwald concludes his book with:

Vaccinations do not protect!

Vaccinations are of no benefit!

Vaccinations are harmful! (Buchwald, page 297).

Vaccinations are big business, a business based on fear. Once we understand that there is no reason for this fear, that the only reason we vaccinate our children is because of fear of these allegedly deadly diseases; that ultimately there is nothing to be afraid of; only then will we realize that not only are vaccinations un-necessary, they are positively harmful. They need to be banned.

This point must be repeatedly made; vaccines are unnecessary.

Vaccines are particularly unnecessary against viral diseases because pathogenic viruses do not exist in humans, animals or plants.

There is a huge push on now to vaccinate the entire population against SARS-CoV-2 because of the fomented fear over this virulent virus, which is much more deadly than any other alleged flu virus. Some doctors and scientists are not in favour of this vaccine because it is a novel vaccine never before tested on humans. However, they still reiterate their belief in the principle of vaccinations. I want to stress that all vaccines are dangerous, all of them. There is no safe vaccine. The SARS-CoV-2 vaccines might be particularly toxic, but every vaccine is toxic.

Core Vaccination Belief

The central belief is that disease is an external entity, an invader, a pathogenic microbe, which vaccination prevents. The legal basis for vaccination does not rely upon 'accepted practice' or 'dominant medical opinion' nor on medical hypotheses and dogmas but on the real threat from pathogenic viruses. If viruses cannot be proven to exist, then there is no scientific basis for vaccination, regardless of the dominant opinion in medicine.

Once we accept that we cannot vaccinate against 'viruses', we also have to realise that vaccinations against bacterial diseases such as tuberculosis and tetanus are ineffective because these bacteria do not cause the respective diseases but are merely present when the disease is present in the host organism.

Just because firefighters are present at a fire does not mean that they caused the fire. Just because flies are present on a dung-heap does not mean that they caused the dung-heap. Similarly, microbes—fungi, bacteria, mycobacteria—are present during a disease but are not its cause.

There are no diseases as entities in themselves. Disease is born of us and in us. Germs do not cause disease. There is no scientific basis for vaccination.

Chapter 3

The Biomedical Paradigm

Modern Medicine is not Scientific

Dr Hans-Ulrich Niemitz wrote a paper in 2003 in response to a query from Dr Ryke Geerd Hamer asking him to compare modern allopathic medicine with German New Medicine. He made two central points:

1. Allopathic medicine applies scientific methods such as observation and statistics but "the mere use of scientific method does not qualify an activity to be a science or a person to be a scientist". Allopathic medicine can only quote statistical survival chances to cancer patients.

2. Allopathic medicine with its many hypotheses, or rather, unproven assumptions, is neither a science nor a natural science. It does not have one hypothesis-free theory concerning the biological events taking place in the individual patient. Allopathic medicine is therefore not scientific and is incapable of understanding the mechanism of any cancer or disease.

In contrast, German New Medicine has Five Biological Laws that are "scientific, free of hypotheses and therefore demonstrable . .. An assertion or system of assertions can only be considered scientific if the assertion or assertions can be denied—technically speaking—or can be tested to determine whether or not they are false" (Niemitz, 2003).

Allopathic medicine has a series of hypotheses such as the immune system and metastasis, which one cannot test because they are theories. These theories have acquired the status of dogmas, and the medical professionals revere them as the absolute truth. Nobody has been able to observe the immune system. Nobody has been able to observe cancer cells in the blood stream or in the lymph nodes, yet these are the two suspected means of cancer transmission or metastasis, whereby cancer allegedly transfers from one organ to another.

Peer Review reinforces the Biomedical Paradigm

I always thought that science in general was open to new ideas, and discoveries. Dr Rustum Roy was a materials scientist with over 50 years' experience. He debunked the idea of science being open to new ideas and presciently argued that the next great breakthrough would be in the field of what he called "Whole-Person Medicine" (Roy, 2002).

> From being the champion of discovery and innovation and newness, science as practiced today has become the main religious establishment of the West ... From a deep curiosity about new facts, establishment science has become a "defender of the faith", a conserver of today's theories.

No one denies that that is the purpose of one key element of the system: peer-review. This key procedure can only check new results by examining whether it conforms to the true faith—to the current theory. Indeed peer-review is most accurately characterised as the "paradigm-police".

Peer-review is the process by which a colleague's work is professionally examined. However, as Dr Roy eloquently puts it, how do you test your colleague's work but by "conformity to the true faith", by conformity to the accepted theories and dogmas of the day. By the "paradigm-police", he means that if the new discovery does not accord with current dogma or accepted theory, then it has to be wrong.

Dr Roy states that peer-review has in fact promoted bad science, because it was in accord with existing theories, and has rejected good science because it was counter to existing theories. Dozens of the greatest advances by Nobel laureates and others were initially rejected by the peer-review system.

Scientists hold up Galileo's challenge to dogma with facts, as the quintessence of science. The cardinals who refused to look into the telescope because dogma had it that the moon's surface had to be perfect are scorned as unscientific. This behaviour is now commonplace in the conventional science establishment.

Dr Roy quotes a philosopher (Alfred North Whitehead): "Advance in detail is admitted: fundamental novelty is barred." He adds, "Peer review is the process which enforces this status."

This state of affairs that applies to science in general, most definitely applies to medicine and biology, with its absolute adherence to the Biomedical Paradigm.

Allopathic Medicine is a Cult

Medicine today is not scientific rather is a secular world religion, which is now a cult. Two possible definitions of the word religion are:

1. A set of beliefs, values and practices based on the teaching of a spiritual leader; and

2. A cause, principle or activity pursued with zeal or conscientious devotion.

The Christian religion would correspond to the first definition of the word religion above: a set of beliefs, values and practices based on the teachings of Jesus.

Allopathic medicine would correspond to the second definition of the word religion because its cause is pursued with such tremendous zeal and conscientious devotion by the medical profession and the scientists. So much so, that one can call it a cult. It is a cult because they claim to be scientists and to operate in a scientific manner but cannot escape from their collective belief in the Biomedical Paradigm. Thus, they are unable to change their mind and revise their opinion based on current scientific evidence.

The Biomedical Paradigm treats the body like a clockwork mechanism. If one part of it breaks down, it is replaced, and theoretically, the 'clockwork mechanism' should work like new again. The Biomedical Paradigm is based on this notion of the body as a machine, of disease as the consequence of breakdown of the machine, and of the doctor's task as repair of the machine (Capra, page 118).

The Biomedical Paradigm is the world viewpoint of the medical profession for over 2,500 years. When I finally understood that modern medicine and biology is a cult, I realised the doctors and scientists themselves could never overthrow their belief system.

The Biomedical Paradigm has invented dogmas such as the Germ Theory of Disease, cellular pathology, carcinogens, metastasis, vaccinations, immune system.... The Biomedical Paradigm consists of about 5,000 or so dogmas that have become the sacred scriptures of a new cult, allopathic medicine, controlled by the doctors, scientists and the pharmaceutical industry, and provided with legal protection by our governments.

The word dogma means an authoritative principle, belief, or statement of ideas or opinion, especially one considered true. Any doctor or scientist rejecting any of the dogmas of the Biomedical Paradigm is regarded as an apostate or charlatan, who must be expelled from the cult and ridiculed.

The key dogmas of the Biomedical Paradigm are:

- Germs cause disease: bacteria cause bacterial diseases and viruses cause viral diseases;
- The cell is the basic building block of life in humans, animals and plants;
- Viruses originate in one cell, spread all over the body and then from one person to another;
- Vaccination prevents infectious diseases;
- Vaccination is the most effective tool of medicine;

- Vaccination caused the reduction in the mortality rate from infectious diseases;

- Cancer spreads from one organ to another by a process called metastasis. For example, liver cancer is a common 'metastasis' or secondary cancer after the diagnosis of bowel cancer. However, no one has ever observed cancerous cells travelling from the bowel to the liver via the lymph nodes or blood stream. Metastasis is the key dogma underpinning their theory of cancer.

I could go on and on but this is not necessary. The central dogmas of medicine today are the belief that germs cause disease and the complementary belief that vaccination prevents infectious disease.

Medicine today is a cult, which has appropriated the rites of the Christian religion, specifically those of the Catholic Church.

- The sacred scriptures of the Biomedical Paradigm, which describes all the various dogmas the Doctors must believe replaces the Bible.

- The Germ Theory of Disease is the central dogma of allopathic medicine. Cellular Pathology is a closely associated dogma, which states that infectious diseases originate in one cell, spread from one cell to the other in the body and then spreads from one person to another.

- Vaccinations play the same initiatory role in allopathic medicine as baptism does in Christianity.

- The search for health has replaced the quest for salvation.
- The eradication of viruses and cancers has taken the place of exorcising demons.
- The hope of physical immortality (cloning, genetic engineering) has been substituted for the hope of eternal life.
- Pharmaceuticals have replaced the sacraments of bread and wine.
- Donations to cancer research or AIDS research have taken precedence over donations to the Church.
- The never-ending search for a hypothetical universal vaccine that can save humanity from all its illnesses, replaces the search for the Holy Grail.
- Patients are alienated from their bodies, just as sinners were alienated from their souls.
- The regular medical check-up with our local friendly doctor replaces confession with our parish priest.
- There is an enforced conformity with the medical dogmas contained in the sacred scriptures of the Biomedical Paradigm, and anyone not conforming is branded a charlatan and is defrocked.
- Doctors have replaced priests and female and male nurses have respectively replaced nuns and brothers.

- Vaccination against the phantom SARS-CoV-2 virus may unfortunately be the means by which some of us receive our last rites from allopathic medicine.

Allopathic medicine is a cult, which has hijacked the World with the Corona Crisis; it has been able to hijack our minds because the vast majority of us believe in its central tenets. However, the uncomfortable truth is that the central dogma of the Biomedical Paradigm—The Germ Theory of Disease—is false.

Asclepius was the god of medicine in ancient Greek mythology. The rod of Asclepius, a staff entwined by a snake is a symbol of medicine today. You see the rod of Asclepius on hospitals, health-care companies, pharmacies etc. The Biomedical Paradigm is rooted in Asclepius, the Greek god of medicine.

The Achilles' heel of allopathic medicine—the fatal flaw that will shatter our collective belief in the Biomedical Paradigm—is the fact that there is no scientific evidence proving the existence of viruses. Once this is accepted, the Biomedical Paradigm will be seen for what it is and can be overthrown. We can break the rod of Asclepius, cut off the head of the snake and cast off this enslaving cult, once we understand that pathogenic viruses do not exist.

Chapter 4

Viral Myths

The Spanish Flu

The Spanish Flu killed between 20 and 50 million people worldwide, depending on the sources you read.

If we take the lower figure, this means that at least three times as many people died of the Spanish Flu as lost their lives during the four years of World War 1, "which ended just as the 1918 pandemic was passing its peak" (Shope, 1958).

World War 1 is rightly remembered for the horrific and unnecessary loss of life, with war memorials in every village and town all over the UK and Ireland commemorating those who died. The Spanish Flu killed at least three times as many people as WW1, but there are no memorials to the victims. We have forgotten the victims of the Spanish Flu; we have airbrushed them from history.

The Spanish Flu has provided the justification for the current lockdown measures to prevent a similar death toll from the SARS-CoV-2 virus.

However, a virus did not cause the Spanish Flu. The horrible truth is that the Spanish Flu of 1918 was manmade—caused by vaccines. The Spanish Flu was the greatest iatrogenic—medically induced—epidemic ever in human history. Until now.

The first wave of the worldwide influenza hit Spain first in the spring of 1918. Thus, it was called the Spanish Flu when it subsequently affected other countries. Interestingly, the Spanish press called it the 'French Flu'. The Spanish Flu was unusual in that it struck down the young and healthy with greater intensity than the usual victims of flu, the new-born, the old and the infirm.

A common expression among American soldiers during the First World War was that "more soldiers were killed by vaccine shots than by shots from enemy guns" (McBean, Chapter 3).

The worst recorded outbreaks of the flu were among soldiers both at the front line and in camps, mostly young and very healthy men. The reason why the outbreaks were worse in the army is because they rigorously enforced vaccinations.

A report from US Secretary of War, Henry L Stimson, confirmed that seven soldiers had dropped dead in an army camp after being vaccinated and that there had been 63 deaths and 28,585 cases of hepatitis as a direct result of the yellow fever vaccine during 6 months of WW1. This yellow fever vaccine was one of 14 to 25 shots given to US soldiers (McBean, Chapter 2).

Many of the returning soldiers from WW1 were insane not from 'shell-shock' but from post-vaccination encephalitis. Vaccines permanently disabled many.

The vaccine manufacturers wanted to continue selling their vaccines to the public after WW1. Their advertising campaigns concerned the dangers posed by 'infected' soldiers returning from far-away lands. The public had to be vaccinated in order to prevent an epidemic on the home front. The tragic irony is that the soldiers were sick from vaccine-induced diseases and the public were encouraged to get more of these vaccines, to prevent the spread of these 'infectious diseases'.

The family of Eleanora McBean refused all vaccinations and remained healthy during the medically induced Spanish Flu. She states that the flu only affected those that had been vaccinated. Because her parents were unvaccinated and were therefore healthy, they were able to look after the sick (McBean, Chapter 2).

If a pathogenic virus had been the cause of the Spanish Flu, surely the McBean family would have been infected? However, the answer by the doctors would be that they must have had a 'strong immune system'. This is one supporting medical dogma to justify another, to explain the impossible within the pattern of thinking of the Biomedical Paradigm.

People were weakened and many died by the cocktail effect from the many different vaccines they had been given. Those who fail to learn from history are condemned to repeat it.[14] Unfortunately, we have not yet officially recognised the true cause of the Spanish Flu. Thus, we are in mortal danger from another catastrophic medically induced epidemic caused by the SARS-CoV-2 vaccines.

The great fear propagated by the virologists, scientists and doctors—prior to COVID-19—was that a novel flu virus

---

14 Quote from Winston Churchill.

would spread from human to human causing a mass pandemic similar to the Spanish Flu of 1918–1920. More people would die because of the increased mobility of humanity through air travel. We should be all afraid of a horrible new virus that could kill more than a 100 million people.

Identifying the Spanish Flu Virus

Dr Jeffrey Taubenberger claims that he reconstructed the Spanish Flu virus from the frozen corpse of a woman who died from it in Alaska in 1918. Dr Taubenberger claims that the bird flu virus H5N1 caused the Spanish flu (Sample, 2005).

The problem with his claim is that there is no scientific paper whereby the Spanish Flu virus was proven to exist in any corpse, because the virus was never isolated. If the virus was not isolated then how can he claim to have produced a genetic model of the virus? Rather than debate the intricacies of how he produced a genetic model of a fictitious virus it would be simpler to ask him to demonstrate how he isolated the virus.

Experiments to Prove that Flu is Contagious

Over the last fifteen years, I have discussed the issue of the 'missing viruses' with many people. The one issue, which prevents people from 'getting it', is the issue of contagion. Most people almost instinctively believe in the existence of viruses, because they assume that they must exist because of their personal experience with the flu or colds and one person in the family infecting others.

I too have had situations in my family where a few of us have had the flu or a bad cold in a close timeframe, which could be explained by contagion. On the other hand, I remember I had a bad flu many years ago and I was off work for a few days, but nobody else in my family got ill or got the flu. I think if people are honest, they too will admit there have been situations where contagion seems to work and other situations where it does not work. However, as human beings, we seem to remember those situations, which confirm our beliefs—so-called confirmation bias—and forget those situations, which we cannot explain because they are contrary to what we would have expected or assumed.

The vast majority of people would assume that the flu is contagious and in particular, that SARS-CoV-2 virus and all its variants are particularly contagious.

Epidemiological evidence claims that the Spanish Flu was particularly virulent and contagious. However, contrary to popular belief, studies on humans during the Spanish Flu failed to prove contagion.

> With all of the observed clinical and epidemiological evidence pointing to the likelihood that the 1918 pandemic influenza was highly contagious and spread from sick to well easily and apparently at the very first available opportunity, one would have anticipated that proof of its contagiousness by transmission tests in human volunteers would have been extremely easy. However, such did not prove to be the case: in not a single controlled experiment was

it possible to demonstrate the transmissibility of the disease.

The most carefully planned and conducted experiments were those carried out by the Navy and the Public Health Service. In the series of experiments conducted in Boston during November and December 1918, 62 volunteers between 15 and 34 years of age were used. Thirty-nine of these had no history of having had influenza at any time, although apparently some degree of exposure had occurred. Filtered and unfiltered secretions from the upper respiratory tracts of patients with typical influenza were sprayed into the nose and throat and instilled into the eyes of some of the volunteers; direct swabbing from nasopharynx to nasopharynx was the method of exposure for others; and in one experiment freshly drawn citrated blood was injected subcutaneously. The results were summarized as follows: "In only one instance was any reaction observed in which a diagnosis of influenza could not be excluded, and here a mildly inflamed throat seemed the more probable cause of the fever and other symptoms. Nothing like influenza developed in the other volunteers."

In an attempt to imitate nature more closely, 10 volunteers were exposed to patients with acute influenza in hospital wards. Each volunteer was placed very near the patient, shook hands with him, chatted with him for 5 minutes and

> then received the patient's breath full in his face five times while he inhaled. Finally the patient coughed five times directly in the subject's face. Each volunteer did this with each of 10 different patients, all of them acutely ill for not more than 3 days. All patients used had typical acute cases selected from a distinct focus or outbreak of disease. None of the volunteers developed the disease (Shope, 1958).

Dr Milton J Rosenau, was one of the authors of the paper "Experiments upon volunteers to determine the cause and mode of spread of influenza, Boston, November and December 1918". His comments are revealing: (Yong, 2020).

- "I think we must be very careful not to draw any positive conclusions from the negative results of this kind. Many factors must be considered. Our volunteers may not have been susceptible. They may have been immune."
- "We entered the outbreak with a notion that we knew the cause of the disease, and were quite sure we knew how it was transmitted from person to person."
- "Perhaps, if we have learned anything, it is that we are not quite sure what we know about the disease."

The HIV Virus

According to the virologists and the doctors, the HIV virus causes AIDS (Acquired Immune Deficiency Syndrome), or a breakdown in our immune system.

The concept of the immune system was invented in the early 1970s to explain why some people are susceptible to disease/cancer, whereas others are not.

The immune system has been presented to us as a type of army in our body whose job is to eventually destroy the malignant cancer cells and malignant germs (Hamer, page 126).

The belief in an immune system is a supporting dogma, which is necessary to explain why the Germ Theory of Disease dogma does not always work. If someone is exposed to a number of people with the flu and does not get sick, this would be deemed to be because of a strong immune system. The immune system dogma is a necessary refinement of the Germ Theory of Disease dogma: One dogma to explain another dogma in order to justify the unexplainable within the pattern of thinking dominating medicine.

If there is no such thing as the immune system then there is certainly no such thing as AIDS or Acquired Immune Deficiency Syndrome. Our body does not suddenly become susceptible to diseases caused by a new virus called HIV.

The HIV virus supposedly occurs in many body fluids, and its transmission, especially in semen and blood to a new person, triggers a slow but inexorable progression to AIDS and finally death (Lanka, 1995).

The HIV retrovirus is the alleged cause of AIDS. A retrovirus belongs to the viral family *Retroviridae*. A retrovirus is simply a particular type of virus.

AIDS was discovered in June 1981 when the CDC (Centre for Disease Control and Prevention) in the US reported a cluster of Pneumocystis carinii pneumonia in five homosexual men in Los Angeles. Initially, it was thought to be exclusively related to homosexual men, hence its original name GRID (Gay Related Immune Deficiency). It is important to stress that just five homosexual men presented with Pneumocystis carinii pneumonia and the hunt was on for a new virus.

In 1982, the CDC introduced the term AIDS to describe this newly invented syndrome because AIDS did not affect just homosexuals.

Because of this belief in the Germ Theory of Disease, the race was on to find the virus that caused AIDS. In 1983, Luc Montagnier led a team of scientists at the Pasteur Institute in France that allegedly discovered the HIV virus. However, he did not isolate the HIV-virus.

If Luc Montagnier had isolated the HIV virus, it should be possible to photograph the isolated HIV virus with an electron microscope. It should then be possible to compare the virus observed in this photograph with the virus as it exists in cells, body fluids or cell cultures in order to distinguish them from other cellular particles which look like viruses but are not viruses (Lanka, 1995).

If the HIV virus exists, it should be possible to biochemically characterise it. The biochemical characterisation would involve separating and photographing the proteins that make up the viral coat surrounding the virus. This produces a pattern, which is characteristic of a particular virus. A similar biochemical characterisation procedure must be carried out for the core of the virus—the virus genome. A good analogy of a biochemical characterisation would be that of a viral fingerprint.

Nobody has produced any such definitive evidence for the existence of the HIV virus nor of any other virus. There are no photographs in existence of an isolated HIV virus. The photographs that have been presented are photographs of virus-like particles in cell cultures, but not of the isolated HIV virus.

The only basis on which the HIV virus is believed to exist is because of an international scientific consensus, which is formed because of their collective belief in the Germ Theory of Disease.

AIDS is defined as a collection of separate diseases such as:

- Pneumocystis carinii pneumonia;
- Kaposi's sarcoma;
- Toxoplasmosis;
- Tuberculosis;
- Clinical symptoms such as extreme weight loss and wasting, exacerbated by diarrhoea, which can be experienced by up to 90% of HIV patients worldwide;
- Meningitis and other brain infections;
- Fungal infections;
- Syphilis; and
- Malignancies such as lymphoma and cervical cancer.

The HIV theory of AIDS is that HIV causes Acquired Immune Deficiency (AID) by destruction of the T4 lymphocytes. AID then leads to the development of the clinical syndrome AIDS, with the above various diseases.

To solve the AIDS conundrum, we have to identify the causes of these separate diseases.

In sub-Saharan Africa, the doctors rarely test for HIV antibodies because it is too costly. They diagnose AIDS by a combination of clinical symptoms such as chronic fevers, diarrhoeas, coughs and weight loss (Lanka, 1995). In reality, these symptoms are diseases of poverty.

One would treat a group of sub-Saharan Africans diagnosed with AIDS for the respective separate diseases that make up AIDS. The 'treatment' in nearly all of these cases would be to provide clean water, good food and hygienic conditions. These Africans would be assured that they do not have AIDS because the HIV virus does not exist. The result of this experiment would be to prove conclusively that AIDS is a name given to a collection of separate diseases and that in the case of sub-Saharan Africa they are usually diseases associated with extreme poverty.

Unlike Africa, the cause of AIDS diseases in the Western world, such as Kaposi's sarcoma is more complex in the case of Western homosexuals. However, one thing for sure is that not one of these diseases is caused by the HIV-virus.

There are a number of inconsistencies about AIDS:

- When the HIV virus was first discovered, it was predicted that AIDS would infect a large percentage of the heterosexual population of the developed world as it has subsequently done in sub-Saharan Africa. This never happened.

- In the Western world, the AIDS virus has predominantly affected two groups: homosexuals and drug-users. Why are heterosexuals in sub-Saharan Africa predominantly affected by AIDS but not in the developed world? People such as President Mbeki of South Africa made this point. How can the same virus affect one population group in the Western world and a different population group in Africa? The doctors and scientists explain this by saying that the HIV retrovirus mutates, but this explanation defies common sense and logic.
- How come people have been diagnosed as HIV-positive and have lived for a long time but have not developed AIDS? The explanation offered will be that they have a strong immune system. This is a circular argument, which is impossible to falsify.
- How come people that were previously diagnosed as HIV-positive have had their diagnosis reversed and are now deemed to no longer have the HIV virus? It just disappeared!

The Reason for AIDS in Sub-Saharan Africa

The reason for AIDS in sub-Saharan Africa is because most people do not have clean drinking water, effective sanitation and adequate food. The remedy for the situation in Africa is to ensure that the people get clean water, effective sanitation and are not malnourished.

Kampala is the capital of Uganda. Many of the poorer people live in a flood zone. There are "heaps of unclaimed garbage" strewn around these houses. During the floods, this rubbish is swept away into the river. There are basic toilets in these areas built above water streams. This raw sewage is released into the streams, the same streams that people use for drinking water. Those that do not have access to these basic toilet facilities use "flying toilets"; they defecate into a plastic bag and throw it into the stream. There are stagnant water holes around these shantytowns in the flood zones, which provide a good breeding ground for mosquitoes. According to the Ugandan National Water and Sewage Corporation, in 2003, only 55% of Kampala was provided with treated water and only 8% with effective sewage disposal (Scheff, 2015).

The situation is not much better in rural areas. Most have no clean water. They wash clothes, bathe and dump their sewage upstream and downstream from where they get their drinking water. Water wells are shared with animals, which being animals, defecate and urinate there (Scheff, 2015).

This description of life in Uganda describes a perfect breeding ground for disease. Instead of tagging clinical symptoms in Kampala such as chronic diarrhoea, weight loss, dysentery, or cholera as being symptomatic of AIDS and then causing further misery to these people by pushing them anti-retroviral drugs, one should initiate a plan for clean drinking water, proper sanitation and adequate food.

The Reason for AIDS in the Developed World

Any homosexual presenting to a doctor with Kaposi's sarcoma and pneumonia will be told that they have Acquired Immune Deficiency Syndrome (AIDS) caused by the phantom HIV virus. The fact that they have these two separate diseases will be regarded as proof that their immune system has broken down.

In the original cases of the handful of homosexuals who presented with both Kaposi's sarcoma and pneumonia, the doctors believed that a new virus must be the causal factor behind these two separate diseases. The search was on for this new virus, which is why the HIV virus was invented.

Instead of the phantom HIV virus, the true cause of these separate diseases was the life-style of the men concerned. Apparently, the original cohort of homosexual men who presented with both pneumonia and Kaposi's sarcoma had a common lifestyle. They took drugs at the weekend to keep them awake, and capable of partying non-stop, and having sex with multiple partners. They then took other drugs to enable them to function during the working week.

Intravenous drug users do not eat enough food and generally have extremely bad living conditions. All their energies are devoted to getting money to support their drug-habit. It is not too difficult to imagine that they are susceptible to various diseases, which would indicate a breakdown of the immune system and they would be deemed to be HIV-positive by the doctors.

The AIDS Tests

HIV-positive is an abbreviation for HIV-antibody positive. The HIV test is performed upon a specimen of the patient's blood where it registers the presence of antibodies. The HIV test is used to verify if these antibodies are caused by the presence of the HIV virus.

If so, they are called HIV antibodies and the patient is said to be HIV positive.

The AIDS test allegedly detects antibodies produced by the immune system in response to infection by the HIV virus. However, how can there be a reliable antibody test for the existence of the HIV virus if the HIV virus itself has never been proven to exist?

The leaflet on an AIDS test kit eloquently proves this point:

> The test for the existence of antibodies against AIDS-associated virus is not diagnostic for AIDS and AIDS-like diseases. Negative test results do not exclude the possibility of contact or infection with the AIDS-associated virus. Positive test results do not prove that someone has AIDS or pre-AIDS disease status nor that he will acquire it (Lanka, 1995).

In other words, the AIDS tests are worthless.

Pathogenic Viruses are Viral Myths

The Germ Theory of Disease was well established and accepted by the time of World War 1 (1914-1918). The soldiers were rigorously vaccinated. Consequently, they were poisoned by the toxic contents of the vaccines. Some died and others were permanently damaged from what was retrospectively called 'shell-shock'. Rather than admit that the cause of these new diseases was vaccines, the doctors and scientists called it the Spanish Flu. More recently, the doctors diagnosed Gulf War Syndrome to cover up vaccine damage.

When the soldiers returned home from WW1, the civilian population were also vaccinated. Despite the excessively high toll from the vaccines, the doctors continued to believe in the necessity and efficacy of vaccines, as did most ordinary people.

The Spanish Flu highlights the importance and significance of these beliefs. Most people believed in the Germ Theory of Disease and therefore willingly accepted the vaccines to prevent infectious diseases. The doctors continued to believe in it despite the high death and sickness toll from those they vaccinated.

Vaccines caused the Spanish Flu, not a fictitious virus. Experiments to prove the contagiousness of the Spanish Flu failed. A phantom virus, a virus that does not exist cannot be contagious.

There is a long-established scientific tradition that those who propose theories provide the proof. According to scientific tradition, it is up to the HIV protagonists to come up with proof that the HIV retrovirus exists. They should be able to cite the scientific publication, which provides conclusive proof that the HIV virus exists. However, there is no such publication.

In 2020, there was no pandemic caused by the phantom SARS-CoV-2 virus because worldwide, there were no excess deaths. In some countries, there was a small increase in deaths and in other countries a small decrease. Overall, there was no pandemic. There were no excess deaths per year—say double or treble the normal death rate. The real pandemic, the pandemic that we are about to endure will be caused by those taking the vaccines. The real pandemic will be the excess death rate and illnesses caused by vaccines, similar to what happened with the Spanish Flu.

Bacteria do exist. They have been isolated, their dimensions measured and photographed. However, there is no such evidence proving the existence of viruses. If they did exist, it would be possible to isolate them. The word isolate means to 'separate something from other things with which it is connected or mixed'. For example, if someone has SARS-CoV-2, and his phlegm is analysed in a laboratory, it should be possible to isolate the virus from all the other constituents of the phlegm. However, it is not possible.

To quote the famous literary detective Sherlock Holmes: "When you eliminate all other possibilities, what remains, no matter how improbable, is the answer." The answer, no matter how improbable, is that the SARS-CoV-2 virus does not exist. It does not cause the collection of symptoms referred to as COVID-19, rather other factors must be the causal agents.

The Spanish Flu, the belief in contagion, the belief in the existence of the HIV-AIDS, SARS-CoV-2 and all other alleged viruses are viral myths.

The Achilles' Heel of the Biomedical Paradigm

The Achilles' Heel of the Biomedical Paradigm is the fact that there is no scientific evidence proving the existence of viruses. There is no evidence substantiating the existence of any alleged virus such as SARS-CoV-2, HIV, mumps, measles, rubella, H1N1 (bird-flu), H5N1 (swine-flu), ebola, zika...If viruses existed, it would be possible to isolate them. Nobody has every isolated any alleged pathogenic virus. Bacteriophages have been isolated, their dimensions measured, photographed and biochemically characterised. Bacteriophages have the same dimensions as all alleged viruses. If it is possible to isolate bacteriophages, why is it not possible to isolate viruses?

Once it is accepted that viruses cannot exist, the Germ Theory of Disease will be understood to be wrong. There will be no need for vaccinations. There will be no more lockdowns because of fictitious viruses. All the dogmas that comprise the Biomedical Paradigm can then be swiftly jettisoned. This will make space for a new understanding of life, health and disease.

It's easier to fool people than to convince them they have been fooled.

Mark Twain, (American writer, 1835–1910)

All great Truths begin as blasphemies.

George Bernard Shaw, (Irish playwright, 1856–1950)

In a time of universal deceit, telling the Truth is a revolutionary act.

George Orwell, (English writer, 1903–1950)

If there is anything that human history demonstrates, it is the extreme slowness with which the academic and critical mind acknowledges facts to exist that present themselves as wild facts, with no staff or pigeonhole, or as facts that threaten to break up the accepted system.

William James (American philosopher, 1842-1910)

In the sciences, people quickly come to regard as their own personal property that which they have learned and had passed on to them at the universities and academies. If someone else comes along with new ideas that contradict the Credo and in fact even threaten to overturn it, then all passions are raised against this threat and no method is left untried to suppress it. People resist it in every way possible: pretending not to have heard about it; speaking disparagingly of it, as if it were not even worth the effort of looking into the matter. And so a new truth can have a long wait before finally being accepted.

Johann Wolfgang von Goethe (German writer, 1749-1832)

Theories of science must be judged on the basis of fact and reason, not by the authority of dogma.

The great tragedy of Science—the slaying of a beautiful hypothesis by an ugly fact.

Thomas Huxley (English biologist, 1825-1895)

Chapter 5

Viruses Cannot Exist

The Burden of Proof for the Existence of Pathogens

In science, if you make an assertion, for example, if you claim that the SARS-CoV-2 virus exists, then you are duty-bound to prove it. The burden of proof is always on the scientist who makes a scientific claim. The burden of proof is not on the reader of the scientific paper to disprove it. Science can only effectively work when the scientist who makes a scientific claim can publicly prove it and other scientists can reproduce the experiment. Once other scientists have verified it, one can then accept that the claim is true.

The general principle is that whoever makes an assertion whether a scientist or a prosecutor, they are duty bound to prove it. The scientists and doctors who state that viruses exist should prove their existence. Analogously, in a court of law, the defense does not have to prove the accused is innocent, rather it is the prosecution, who claim that the defendant is guilty that are obliged to prove it.

A scientist cannot employ the 'Martian argument', which states that Martians exist because there is no proof that they do not exist. You cannot prove a negative; you cannot prove that Martians do not exist. However, you can at the very least expect that anyone who states with certainty that they exist to provide the evidence.

Corn-circles (flattened corn in the shape of a circle) in a large cornfield could provide indirect evidence of the landing of a UFO. Unless you have direct evidence for the existence of the UFO, indirect evidence such as corn-circles does not prove its existence, no matter if there are thousands of such corn-circles. If you already have direct evidence for the existence of an UFO, then one could legitimately use indirect evidence such as corn-circles to prove the existence of an UFO.

Citing indirect evidence for the existence of a pathogenic virus is not sufficient to prove its existence. Before we rely on any indirect evidence for the existence of viruses, the virologists should have directly proven that the virus exists.

Proving that Germs (Bacteria and Viruses) are Pathogens

The German pathologist Friedrich Gustav Jacob Henle (1809–1885) first formulated the following postulates, which the German bacteriologist Robert Koch (1843–1910) later modified. The postulates are called Koch's postulates or the Henle-Koch postulates. They establish the four necessary criteria to confirm that a pathogen is the cause of a specific infectious disease.

Henle-Koch Postulates

1. The pathogenic microbe (bacteria or virus) can be observed in the body fluids of a host suffering from the disease. This pathogen is not present in a healthy host.

2. The pathogen can be isolated from the diseased host and cultured in the laboratory.

3. The cultured pathogen causes the same disease when introduced into another host.

4. The pathogen can be re-isolated from that experimentally infected host.

The theory behind these postulates is logical and easily understood. You can observe pathogens in the body fluids of an infected host; you can isolate them from the host and grow or culture them in the laboratory; you can inject them into another host and cause the same disease and you can then re-isolate the same pathogen from the newly infected host. These postulates or criteria, if fulfilled, would prove that a specific pathogen causes a specific disease.

Bacteria & the Henle-Koch Postulates

If a patient is suffering from tuberculosis, it is possible to see tubercular bacteria (mycobacterium tuberculosis MTB) in a tissue sample. One cannot see the tubercular bacteria in a healthy patient. Thus, tubercular bacteria satisfy the first postulate.

It is possible to purify tubercular bacteria and culture them in the laboratory thus fulfilling the second postulate.

Guinea pigs were injected with mycobacterium MTB to test the third postulate but it failed to cause tuberculosis in the guinea pigs and they were fine (Widmer, page 44).

The third postulate could be tested on humans by introducing the mycobacterium tuberculosis MTB into a healthy subject in order to cause tuberculosis to occur in that previously healthy patient. If I were to drink or breathe in a huge quantity of mycobacterium tuberculosis MTB isolated from somebody with tuberculosis, I would not get this disease. I would bet that if 1,000 people fully understood that they are not pathogens, and drank or inhaled or otherwise ingested huge quantities of purified tubercular bacteria, not one of them would get tuberculosis. Tubercular bacteria do not cause tuberculosis; rather, they are present when the patient has tuberculosis.

Bacteria do exist but they are not transmissible from one person to another and cause the same disease; there is no contagion for bacteria. Bacteria fail the third postulate because they are not pathogenic. Moreover, vaccinations against bacterial microbes are not necessary because they are not pathogenic; they are not contagious.

Viruses & the Henle-Koch Postulates

Viruses fail the first postulate because no one has ever seen or photographed a virus in a bodily fluid from a human or animal (Lanka, 2020:3).

Currently, electron microscopes have a resolution of 0.2nm. The alleged diameter of pathogenic viruses varies between 20nm to 200nm. If viruses did exist, it would be possible to view them using an electron microscope. Thus, Dr Lanka authoritatively states that nobody has ever seen a virus in a bodily fluid from a human or animal. The electron micrographs of viruses show normal cellular particles from dying tissues and cells (Lanka, 2020:1). They are not photographs of isolated viruses.

Nevertheless, even if one accepted that what the virologists observe in the electron microscope is actually a virus, one should be able to isolate it. However, there is no scientific paper available, which demonstrates the isolation of a virus. Thus, viruses fail the second postulate.

What is a Virus?

Scientists postulated the existence of viruses in the late 1800s before it was technically possible to prove their existence.

If someone had a fever, and bacteria were present—they were deemed the cause. If they had a fever and the doctors could not observe any bacteria, then they would have suspected that viruses were the causal agent. This is all perfectly understandable if one believes in the Germ Theory of Disease.

The received wisdom is that pathogenic viruses are poisonous microscopic entities that invade a host cell, multiply uncontrollably, invade other cells, spread throughout the body, and are transmissible between people and animals. These viruses are so pathogenic that they can even kill the host.

Until 1952, the virologists believed that a virus was a toxic protein or enzyme. They carried out two control experiments, which conclusively proved that their assumption was wrong and that a virus could not be a toxic protein. Firstly, they never observed a toxic protein in an electron microscope. They observed no difference between the electron microscope photographs from healthy people and those infected with the virus. Secondly, when healthy tissue was decaying, it produced proteins, which were the exact same as those from tissue that had been 'infected' by a virus; thus, there were no toxic proteins (Lanka, 2020:3).

Nonetheless, the vaccination programme continued apace against viruses, even though the scientists did not know what a virus was and had abandoned the idea of it being a toxic protein. They simply 'knew' that a virus had to exist because of their firm belief in the Germ Theory of Disease.

Bacteriophages

The virologists had to come up with a new concept of what a virus was. Molecular genetics came to the fore in the early 1950s. They invented the idea that a virus had to be a pathogenic gene. The model for the 'virus-gene' in humans, animals and plants, which developed from 1953 onwards was a bacteriophage. Scientists first discovered bacteriophages in 1915. Electron microscopes were applied in research laboratories from 1938 and thus the bacteriophages could be photographed (Lanka, 2020:1).

There are thousands of different types of phages. Bacteriophages of one type always have the same structure. They consist of a molecule, comprised of nucleic acid, which is enwrapped by a protein shell of a given number and composition. In simple terms, a phage is comprised of a nucleic acid core enwrapped by a protein shell (Lanka, 2015:1).

This effect of the formation of phages does not occur with pure bacteria extracted from the environment. When nutrients are withdrawn from the bacteria, or when their living conditions become impossible, normal bacteria—bacteria not grown in the laboratory—create known survival forms called spores, which can live for a long time or even eternally. As soon as the living conditions improve, bacteria re-emerge from these spores. Thus, one can say that spores emanate from healthy bacteria when the living conditions become impossible. Conversely, when the environment improves, bacteria re-emerge from these spores (Lanka, 2015:1).

Isolated bacteria or bacteria grown in a laboratory lose their characteristics and abilities over time. Many of them do not die off automatically through this inbreeding but rather turn into smaller particles called bacteriophages. When bacteriophages were first discovered, the scientists initially believed they were 'bacterial viruses' or 'bacteria-eaters' (Lanka, 2015:1).

They then subsequently discovered that phages were not 'bacteria eaters' but that they emerge from bacteria when the living conditions rapidly deteriorate and that bacteria remerge from phages once the living conditions improve. In other words, there is a symbiotic relationship between bacteria and bacteriophages, similar to bacteria and spores. Bacteriophages is an incorrect term. They are not 'bacteria eaters', rather they should be regarded as mini spores and the building blocks of bacteria. The scientists use the known structure of bacteriophages as a model for all alleged human and animal viruses (Lanka, 2015:1).

It is possible to purify phages using density gradient centrifugation. The isolated phages can then be biochemically characterised. This is essential for identifying the specific type of phage. The isolate consisting of the purified phages is divided in two. One part is used to determine the size, type and composition of the nucleic acid. The second part is used to determine the number, size and morphology of the proteins. University biology students study and perform these standard simple techniques. Scientists have proven the existence of over two thousand different types of bacteriophages in this manner. If any alleged pathogenic virus existed, it would be possible to prove their existence by this method (Lanka, 2015:1).

Pathogenic Viruses

Bacteriophages have been purified, photographed and biochemically analysed—both the nucleic acid and the protein shell. If any alleged pathogenic virus existed, it would be possible to purify it using density gradient centrifugation and to then biochemically analyse it. It has not occurred to the virologists that no alleged pathogenic virus has ever been purified and biochemically analysed in a similar manner to phages.

The virologists believe that a pathogenic virus is similar in composition and structure to a bacteriophage and that the genetic material of a pathogenic virus is comprised of either DNA or RNA. They believe that the coronavirus and the measles virus consist of an RNA molecule enwrapped by a protein shell.

Marine Brown Alga Ectocarpus siliculosus Virus

Dr Stefan Lanka was born in 1963. He studied marine biology at university because he wanted to learn more about the mystery of life.

During his undergraduate years, Dr Lanka studied a 'virus' that had 'infected' a sea alga. The virus did not make the sea-alga sick. In fact, the virus helped the sea alga to thrive, which was quite the opposite of what he had expected. He was excited, because he then believed that he had discovered the first stable non-pathogenic 'virus-host' relationship. The virus did not threaten the host and both co-existed harmoniously or endo-symbiotically.

In order to prove the existence of this virus, he isolated, photographed and biochemically characterised it. The photograph was taken by an electron microscope invented in the 1930s and the biochemical characterisation was carried out using techniques invented in the 1970s.

Dr Lanka had discovered the Marine Brown Alga Ectocarpus siliculosus virus. It is referred to a 'giant virus'. This giant virus is not pathogenic and enables the Marine Brown Alga Ectocarpus siliculosus to thrive because of, and not despite it.

Giant viruses only exist in simple life forms such as fibre algae, a particular type of a unicellular chlorella algae. In these simple life forms, they are not poisonous but perform a useful and necessary function. They are not harmful in any way to the host organism. Rather, they are beneficial and enable the host organism to thrive in their presence.

The Marine Brown Alga Ectocarpus siliculosus virus reproduces itself in the algae, can leave the algae and reproduce itself again in other algae of this kind, without having any negative effects. The sea algae continue to bloom and flourish in the presence of this virus. Dr Lanka published a scientific paper documenting this in 1990.

The reason why he initially called it a 'virus' was because it had all the characteristics of a virus. It has a genome at its core surrounded by a protein shell. It is important to note that Dr Lanka would not use the word virus today because it has pathogenic or disease-inducing connotations, but would instead use the word 'biont', which means living organism.

Density Gradient Centrifugation

Density Gradient Centrifugation was developed in the 1950s. It is now the standard method for the purification of bionts—such as bacteriophages and giant viruses. Bacteriophages range between 25nm–200nm in diameter and have a similar size to all alleged pathogenic viruses.

The liquid containing the bacteriophages is applied on another inert liquid already in the test tube. The inert liquid in the test-tube is gradient layered, with a high concentration at the bottom of the test tube and a low concentration at the top of the test tube. The test tube with the bacteriophages is then spun or centrifuged and all the particles are fixed in the test tube according to their density. This is why this process is called Density Gradient Centrifugation (Lanka, 2015:1).

The layer where many particles of the same density gather becomes 'cloudy' and is called a 'band'. The phages in a band can be removed with a pipette. The extracted concentrated phages are an isolate. An electron micrograph can confirm the presence of phages in the isolate. This photograph will also be an indication for the purity of the isolate, if it shows no other particles but the phages. The appearance and the diameter of the phages can also be determined with the help of the micrograph (Lanka, 2015:1).

Despite the fact that the microbiology manuals refer to Density Gradient Centrifugation as the 'virus isolation technique', it is not used in experiments to demonstrate the existence of pathogenic viruses (Lanka, 2015:1).

If bacteriophages can be purified using Density Gradient Centrifugation, it ought to be possible to purify any alleged pathogenic virus, because the virologists believe they have similar dimensions to those of bacteriophages.

Proving the Existence of a Pathogenic Virus

How do you prove that something, which does not exist, such as a pathogenic virus, does not actually exist? On the face of it, it appears to be a stupid, if not a pointless task. Moreover, it would appear to be intrinsically impossible to prove a negative.

However, when you ask the virologists what a pathogenic virus is, then you can at least construct an experiment to determine whether it exists according to their belief of what it is. The virologists believe that all pathogenic viruses that affect humans, animals and plants are similar to bacteriophages. Scientists, biologists, virologists and medical doctors believe that all alleged pathogenic viruses have a nucleic acid at their core—whether DNA (DeoxyriboNucleic Acid) or RNA (RiboNucleic Acid)—surrounded by a protein shell.

Thus, the virologists claim that pathogenic viruses are similar to phages and 'giant viruses'. If one applies the same criteria to all alleged pathogenic viruses as one does to phages and giant viruses, there would be four steps involved in proving the existence of a pathogenic virus.

It must be:

1. Isolated;
2. Photographed;
3. Dimensions Measured; and
4. Biochemically Characterised.

In order to identify a virus definitively, one would have to isolate it. It must be isolated from the cells, body fluids or cell culture and above all it must be freed from contaminants. They can be easily separated from other cellular components because of their weight and/or sedimentation characteristics using density gradient centrifugation. It does not matter what the virus is isolated from, whether from body fluids, cell cultures, plasma or serum: Once isolated, a pure virus is seen regardless of where it comes from.

Secondly, the isolated virus must be photographed with an electron microscope.

Thirdly, its dimensions must be measured.

Fourthly, the proteins making up the viral coat are separated from each other and photographed. They are separated in an electrical field according to their size. This produces a pattern, which is characteristic of the type of virus. A similar separation and identification procedure must be carried out for the DNA or RNA at the core of the virus. It is legitimate to speak of a new virus only after the viral proteins and nucleic acid components have been properly identified. This process is called the biochemical characterisation of the virus.

One can only prove the existence of a pathogenic virus when one has documented these four steps.

Indirect Evidence for the Existence of a Virus

Nobody has ever isolated any alleged pathogenic virus, neither the measles virus not the SARS-CoV-2 virus. Nobody has ever directly proven the existence of any alleged pathogenic virus.

Instead, the scientists and medical doctors use indirect methods to prove the existence of viruses. Three indirect methods are currently used to identify the presence of a virus: diagnosis of a viral infection, antibody testing and a PCR test.

a) Diagnosis of viral infection

Doctors diagnose a viral infection by clinical symptoms such as fever, high temperature, sweating etc. Thus, doctors do not diagnose viral infections by directly identifying the virus rather they assume that a virus must be the underlying cause of the symptoms.

b) Antibody testing

According to the UK Department of Health and Social Care:

> Antibody tests are used to detect antibodies to the COVID-19 virus to see if it is likely that you have previously had the virus. The test works by taking a blood sample and testing for the presence of antibodies to see if you have developed an immune response to the virus.[15]

The obvious question is how can you detect antibodies to a phantom virus? If you cannot prove the existence of any virus, the antibody tests for the respective viruses are by definition meaningless.

c) PCR Test

The paper "Detection of 2019 novel coronavirus (2019-nCoV) by real-time RT-PCR", explains how scientists detect the alleged new coronavirus—SARS-CoV-2. This PCR method is an indirect method for the detection of viruses, without having isolated or purified the virus in the first place. They explicitly admit this in the paper with confessional phrases such as "without having virus material available" and "as virus isolates are unavailable".

In simple terms, they detect RNA strands from what they believe is the SARS-CoV-2 virus, which they believe shares the same RNA sequences with the SARS coronavirus. The problem with all of this is that they have never isolated the SARS coronavirus, the SARS-CoV-2 virus nor indeed any other alleged virus.

---

15 https://www.gov.uk/government/publications/coronavirus-covid-19-antibody-tests/coronavirus-covid-19-antibody-tests Retrieved March 2021.

What they are doing with RT-PCR is they are detecting strands of RNA and arbitrarily determining that they belong to the suspected novel coronavirus, without ever having isolated the novel coronavirus in the first place. The science behind all of this is demonstrably wrong. They are attempting to come up with the genome sequence of viruses by stringing fragments of nucleic acids strands together, which they believe belong to the virus. They form a consensus on what fragments of nucleic acids (RNA) belongs to the novel coronavirus. All of this, without ever having isolated the novel coronavirus in the first place.

Barden vs Lanka: The Measles Virus Case (2012-2017)

In November 2011, Dr Stefan Lanka offered €100,000 to anyone who could prove the existence of the measles virus. He got the idea of the prize from a senior state prosecutor in order to establish in the subsequent civil trial that there is no scientific evidence proving the existence of the measles virus. The rationale for the prize was to prevent the planned compulsory measles vaccination in Germany, which was finally implemented in March 2020 (Lanka 2020:1).

The conditions of the prize were that the scientific paper had to be published by the Robert Koch Institute, which is the responsible body in Germany for the identification of pathogenic viruses (Lanka 2020:1).

Dr David Bardens presented six scientific papers, which he claimed proved the existence of the measles virus (Lanka, 2015:1).

Paper 1: John F Enders, Thomas C Peebles
Propagation in tissue cultures of cytopathogenic agents from patients with measles
(Proc Soc Exp Biol Med. 1954 Jun; 86 (2): 277–286)

Paper 2: Bech V, Magnus Pv
Studies on measles virus in monkey kidney tissue cultures. Acta Pathol Microbiol Scand. 1959; 42 (1): 75–85.

Paper 3: Nakai M, Imagawa DT
Electron microscopy of measles virus replication.
J. Virol. 1969 Feb; 3v (2): 87–97.

Paper 4: Lund GA, Tyrell, DL, Bradley RD, Scraba DG
The molecular length of measles virus RNA and the structural organization of measles nucleocapsids.
J. Gen. Virol. 1984 Sep;65 (Pt 9): 1535–42

Paper 5: Horikami SM, Moyer SA
Structure, Transcription, and Replication of Measles Virus. Curr Top Microbiol Immunol. 1995; 191: 35–50.

Paper 6: Daikoku E, Morita C, Kohno T, Sano K
Analysis of Morphology and Infectivity of Measles Virus Particles. Bulletin of the Osaka Medical College. 2007; 53 (2): 107–14.

Paper 1, 1954, John F Enders, Thomas C Peebles

John Franklin Enders and Thomas Peebles published this paper in June 1954. It is the most important paper regarding the current belief in the existence of the measles virus. In December 1954, John Franklin Enders won the Nobel Prize in medicine along with two other colleagues for their in vitro[16] culture of the poliovirus in 1949. He applied the same technique he used in connection with the poliovirus to the measles virus in his June 1954 paper. Because he won the Nobel Prize for Medicine in December 1954, his method for 'isolating' the polio and measles virus was subsequently accepted as scientific truth.

Enders and Peeble dramatically reduced the nutrient solution and added cell-destroying antibiotics to the cell culture before introducing the allegedly infected fluid containing the 'measles virus'.

The authors misinterpreted the subsequent death of the cells as proof of the presence of and simultaneously as isolation of the measles virus. The authors of the paper did not carry out any control experiments to exclude the possibility that it was the deprivation of nutrients as well as the antibiotics, which led to the death of the cells.

I did not grasp the meaning of this until after many subsequent re-readings. If you add a sterile sample to the cell culture, the cells would die off, as they would with a sample from a child with measles. This control experiment would prove that it was the experimental conditions, which caused the death of the cells and not the presence of the measles virus. The experimental conditions were that the cell culture had reduced nutrients (up to 80% less nutrients to make it more receptive to the 'virus') and was poisoned by antibiotics (to kill off bacteria, so that bacteria could not be claimed to be the cause of the death of the cells).

---

16 In vitro means in glass. It refers to studies performed with microorganisms or cells outside their normal biological context. They are commonly called test-tube studies.

If they had carried out this control experiment, they would have determined that the experimental conditions caused the death of the cells and that the death of the cells had nothing to do with the sample containing the alleged measles virus. This control experiment seems so obvious but the virologists have yet to carry it out.

Paper 2, 1959, Bech V, Magnus Pv

This paper states that the technique used by Enders-Peeble was not suitable for isolating the virus. The virologists have not heeded this paper and have ignored it or swept it under the carpet because it does not fit in with their beliefs. Nonetheless, it is correct. The death of cells in the manner described in paper 1 above occurs with both sterile material and 'infected' material. Thus, the Enders-Peeble paper does not demonstrate the isolation of the measles virus (Lanka, 2015:1).

Paper 3, 1969, Nakai M, Imagawa DT

In the third paper, the authors photographed typical cellular particles inside the cells and misinterpreted them as the measles virus. They did not isolate the measle virus. They failed to determine and describe the biochemical structure of what they were presenting as a virus. They did not apply density gradient centrifugation. They simply centrifuged fragments of dead cells at the bottom of a test tube and then, without describing their biochemical structure, they misinterpreted the cellular debris as viruses (Lanka, 2015:1).

Paper 4 Lund GA, Tyrell, DL, Bradley RD, Scraba DG & Paper 6 Daikoku E, Morita C, Kohno T, Sano K

Papers 4 & 6 present the same situation as above in paper 3. They did not isolate the measles virus (Lanka, 2015:1).

Paper 5, 1995, Horikami SM, Moyer SA

The fifth publication is a review describing the consensus process as to what nucleic acid molecules from the dead cells would represent the genome of the measles virus. The result is that dozens of researchers teams work with short pieces of cell-specific molecules, after which—following a given model—they put all the pieces together on a computer. However, this jigsaw puzzle made of so many pieces was never scientifically proven to exist as a whole intact entity and was never obtained from an isolated virus (Lanka, 2015:1).

This paper describes how the genome of the measles virus is theoretically constructed. Again, how can you recreate the genome of the measles virus, if you have never isolated it in the first place?

Referring to this publication, the court-appointed expert stated that it described the gold standard for the identification of a virus—by determining its genome. However, the expert must not have read the paper because its authors stated that the exact molecular composition and functions of the measles virus genome will have to be the object of further research, which is why they had to rely on other virus models in order to achieve a consensus on the structure of the measles virus (Lanka, 2015:1).

Dr Lanka hired two independent laboratories to investigate the alleged measles virus. The both confirmed that the typical gene sequence of quite normal healthy cells has been wrongly interpreted as central component parts of the 'measles virus'. Short genetic sequences (from normal healthy cells) have been arbitrarily assembled together in order to make up a theoretical model of the 'measles virus', and this is stated to be the genetic model or genome of the measles virus.

The six papers do not prove the existence of the measles virus

As stated above, the Enders-Peeble paper is the most significant of the six papers because it was published in June 1954 and the lead author, John Franklin Enders, won the Nobel Prize for medicine in December 1954. Virologists today believe that this method is a scientific method for the 'isolation' of all viruses, not just the measles virus.

None of these papers used the density gradient centrifugation technique to isolate the measles virus. If they had, they would have failed because the measles virus does not exist.

Legal Proceedings

Dr Bardens urged Dr Lanka to avoid a costly legal dispute and to pay him the prize money. Dr Lanka replied that none of the six publications contained an identifiable virus, rather easily recognizable typical cellular particles and structures (Lanka, 2020:1).

Dr Lanka refused to pay up, because the papers did not prove the existence of the measles virus, neither individually nor collectively. Moreover, the Robert Koch Institute did not publish them.

Dr Bardens began legal proceedings in late 2013 to obtain the €100,000 in prize money. The Ravensburg district court in the German state of Baden-Württemberg ruled in favour of Dr David Bardens in March 2015. Dr Bardens did not even present the six papers to the court, nevertheless, the court ruled in his favour. Presumably, they believed that the measles virus must exist, without having to examine the evidence. Dr Lanka appealed this court decision.

The Baden-Württemberg higher regional court (*Oberlandesgericht OLG*) in Stuttgart on February 2016 overturned the judgment of the Ravensburg court in February 2016 and dismissed the action.

Dr Bardens confessed to the judge during the appeal at the Stuttgart higher regional court that he had never read the six publications. The six publications are significant because they do not assume the prior existence of the measles virus. This is in contrast with over 30,000 technical articles about measles, which assume that the measles virus exists (Lanka, 2020:1).

Dr David Bardens filed an appeal against the judgment of the higher regional court to the German Federal Court of Justice *(Bundesgerichtshof BGH)*. The primary basis of his appeal was his belief that what Dr Lanka factually stated about the 'measles virus' posed a threat to public health. The Federal Court of Justice rejected his position. Thus, it confirmed the judgment of the higher regional court in Stuttgart from 16 February 2016.

The sum of €100,000, which Dr Stefan Lanka had offered as a reward for scientific proof of the existence of the alleged measles virus, did not have to be paid and Dr David Bardens was ordered to bear all legal costs.

Five experts were involved in the case. All five experts, including Professor Andreas Podbielski have stated that none of the six publications provides scientific proof for the existence of the measles virus.

Virology is not scientific

The word science comes from the Latin *scientia* meaning 'knowledge'.

> Science is the intellectual and practical activity encompassing the systematic study of the structure and behaviour of the physical and natural world through observation and experiment.[17]

Scientists should observe professional standards and be aware of all of the developments in his field. All steps of an experiment should be verified by control experiments to ensure that it is not the experiment itself that causes the result. Scientists are supposed to doubt everything and everyone, especially their own ideas. This helps to avoid misinterpretations and undesirable developments.

17 https://www.lexico.com Retrieved March 2021.

Scientists should question what they have learned, and what they teach. They should question existing paradigms or patterns of thinking in their respective field.

The virologists, doctors and other scientists have proven that they are unscientific because they have refused to question the Germ Theory of Disease, which is the central dogma of medicine and biology. For over 30 years, Dr Lanka has repeatedly pointed out that nobody has ever purified any alleged pathogenic virus. It is possible to isolate bionts (bacteriophages and giant viruses), which have a similar size to all alleged pathogenic viruses. He has repeatedly asked the virologists why they cannot isolate any alleged pathogenic virus.

The virologists continue to be obsessed with recreating or sequencing the genome of viruses such as SARS-CoV-2, without ever having isolated the virus in the first place. They are trying to sequence a pathogenic virus, which is a theoretical construct, a phantom, something that they believe exists even though it is not possible to isolate it.

Virology is not scientific. It is completely out of touch with biological reality. We need to go back to the beginning of allopathic medicine and revisit its central dogma. The Germ Theory of Disease is wrong and viruses cannot exist. They cannot exist because no one has ever observed a virus in an electron microscope nor isolated it.

Chapter 6

No Record Exists

Querying the Virologists

In the mid-1980s, Luc Montagnier claimed that he had discovered a new virus—HIV. When Dr Lanka discovered a new non-pathogenic virus in the early-1990s, he was deemed a technical expert, a virologist. He was asked by Professor Fritz Pohl (discoverer of the Z-structure of nucleic acid) to examine the scientific literature on the HIV-virus.

He thoroughly researched it and could not find any scientific publications, where the HIV virus had been isolated. Dr Stefan Lanka could not believe that thousands of researchers were attending international AIDS conferences, despite the fact that there was absolutely no evidence for the existence of the HIV virus. It did not make any sense. He was so dumbstruck by the enormity of his discovery that initially, he could not discuss it with anyone for six months. The implications of his discovery were and still are profound.

He further examined the scientific literature and discovered there also was no scientific evidence for the existence of the mumps, measles and rubella viruses, against which we allow doctors and nurses vaccinate our children.

Dr Lanka had discovered that there was no scientific evidence for the existence of any pathogenic virus.

In fact, the 'viruses' that really do exist are beneficial. He later discovered that in one liter of seawater there are about 100 million 'giant viruses'. He writes sardonically that it is just as well the doctors are not aware of this otherwise, we would all have to wear a total body condom before we go for a sea-swim!

The Germ Theory of Disease states that germs or microbes (bacteria or viruses) from an external source invade the body and are the cause of infectious disease. The concept of bacteria (and subsequently viruses) causing specific diseases became publicly accepted knowledge in the latter part of the 1800s.

Dr Lanka had scientifically determined that these alleged pathogenic viruses could not exist because no scientist has ever seen or isolated them.

Dr Lanka told everybody, but his colleagues and professors were not interested. His professors told him to keep quiet and complete his doctorate. He could not engage the virologists, the scientists and the medical doctors. They were not true scientists willing to test every hypothesis and query their own belief systems.

Together with Karl Krafeld, he initiated the concept of 'citizen enquiry' in late 2000. Their idea was to get ordinary citizens to query the authorities for the scientific proof for the existence of pathogenic viruses.

Most people at these initial meetings expected the authorities to provide this evidence. However, they did not. Ordinary citizens in Germany, Austria and Switzerland, people like you and me, requested from the authorities the scientific proof that pathogenic viruses such as measles, mumps and rubella actually exist. The point about ordinary citizens questioning the authorities was for lay people to understand that the science was demonstrably wrong, that no scientist had ever isolated any alleged pathogenic virus. The idea was for a bottom-up groundswell of people to request the scientific evidence, so much so, that the authorities would be overwhelmed and forced to admit that pathogenic viruses cannot exist. However, to date, the authorities have still not admitted and confessed that this is the case.

When you query the authorities, there are three possible sources, which they can use to 'prove' the existence of pathogenic viruses,

1. Medical textbooks;
2. Photographs of viruses; and
3. Scientific publications.

1 Medical textbooks

A medical textbook is not a scientific work, but a book for teaching accepted truths. A textbook is referred to as a secondary source. A primary source such as a scientific journal provides direct proof for a scientific statement. One can then legitimately refer to these primary sources in a secondary source such as a textbook.

Medical textbooks cannot cite any scientific publications proving the existence of pathogenic viruses, because none exists.

2 Photographs of Viruses

Sometimes the authorities produce photographs of 'viruses'. However, these photographs are not of isolated viruses, but of what the scientists believe to be viruses in wafer-thin tissue slices.

These images are not direct photographs of an isolated virus. The scientists who produced these photographs cannot claim that they are direct photographs of a virus because the virus was not purified before the photograph was taken.

Despite all this, the scientists allege the contrary to the public and claim that these are photographs of viruses. Certainly, my understanding was that these were direct photographs of viruses, as one would normally understand a photograph to be.

How to detect a fraudulent photograph of a virus

There are two easy ways to detect a fraudulent picture of a virus:

A) Read the caption; and

B) Examine the photograph.

A) Read the caption

The caption usually states that the photograph is of cells, which allegedly contain viruses. The caption does not even claim that the virus has been isolated. These photographs show cells and typical cellular substances of all types. Scientists are aware of these structures, which serve functions such as transport inside and outside the cells. Nonetheless, the virologists fraudulently claim that these photographs are of viruses.

B) Examine the Photograph

All bionts (phages and so-called giant viruses) of a particular type always have the same size and shape. If the picture shows a particular virus, but with the virus having different shapes, you immediately know, it is fraudulent and is not a photograph of an isolated virus.

If the photograph is a colour-photograph, you know that it is a fabricated photograph, a CGI—Computer Generated Image—because photographs from an electron microscope are only in black and white.

The virologists believe in the existence of viruses. These alleged virus photographs are what they believe to be 'viruses' contained in a tissue sample. They are not photographs of purified viruses. They know this but fraudulently claim the contrary to the public.

When the virologists, the scientists and the doctors say that these photographs are direct photographs of viruses, they are deliberately lying. There is no other way to put this; they are criminally negligent because they are supporting the enormous scientific fraud that pathogenic viruses exist.

3 Scientific publications

On rare occasions, the authorities cite original scientific publications. Again, these scientific publications invariably describe how a photograph of a wafer-thin size tissue was produced which allegedly contains a virus. However, the putative virus has not been isolated from the tissue sample. If you actually read these scientific publications, they explicitly state that they have not isolated the virus.

The only relevant scientific publication proving the existence of a pathogenic virus is one, which demonstrates:

1. How the virus was isolated;
2. The photograph of the virus in its purified form;
3. How its dimensions were measured; and
4. How, the virus was biochemically characterised, both the core and the coat of the virus.

When you examine the scientific publications, they sometimes use the word 'isolate'. Some of the papers even have the words 'isolate' or 'isolation' in their title, which would imply that they have isolated the virus. However, this is not the case.

David Crowe, a Canadian biologist and citizen journalist, informed me during an interview in June 2018 on his podcast show 'The Infectious Myth' that it was much better to use the word 'purify' instead of the word 'isolate'.[18] This is because the virologists have so abused the meaning of the word isolate as to render it meaningless. Virologists and microbiologists take a swab sample from a patient with 'viral symptoms' and consider that to be 'virus isolation' when it is in reality just mucous. The use of the

18 https://infectiousmyth.podbean.com/e/the-infectious-myth-there-are-no-viruses-with-james-mccumiskey-060518/ Retrieved October 2021

word 'isolation' to describe this mucous, which allegedly contains a virus, does not accord with our general understanding of the word 'isolation'.

> But, they imply and promote the true meaning of the process of isolation, i.e., to obtain something by extraction, purification, and identification, reflected by well-known pretty pictures of the DNA/RNA, proteins, and viruses such as a spherical body with spikes (aka coronavirus).
>
> The virologists' version of the definition is incorrect and causing the problem. Wherever one looks for the virus, one always finds a suffix with it, e.g., "virus isolate," "virus culture," "virus lysate," etc., (which are soups, mixtures or gunks), never "virus" alone; however, it is presented and promoted as pure "virus."
>
> The made-up definition of "virus-isolation" makes the story of the SARS-CoV-2 virus, its infection, and pandemic very clear, i.e., nothing is real about them, but all are fake. No one has seen the virus, found it, or isolated it as claimed. It is all bogus (Qureshi, 2021).

This is why I now use the words 'purification' or 'purify" instead of 'isolation' or 'isolate'.

Initial Correspondence with the Virologists

In early 2006, I decided to take up the 'citizen enquiry' challenge in Ireland initially and then the UK. I contacted the politicians, the Minister for Health, the Irish Prime Minister, other politicians and journalists, questioning the existence of pathogenic viruses. This was a fruitless endeavour, a waste of time and energy. They all relied on expert scientific opinion. I then focussed my attention on those people I perceived were the relevant technical experts.

For example, I contacted Dr Darina O'Flanagan MD, who was the then director of the HPSC (Health Protection Surveillance Centre). The HPSC was established in 1998 and was formerly known as the National Disease Surveillance Centre (NDSC). It monitors and reports on vaccine uptake and effectiveness. It was for this reason that I contacted Dr Darina O'Flanagan MD. She responded promptly the same day to my first email in March 2006 and provided me with the names of two textbooks, which allegedly contained the primary references proving the existence of the mumps, measles and rubella viruses.

> I recommend Mandell Bennett and Dolin on Principles and Practices of infectious diseases. You will find plenty of primary references in there.
>
> I recommend Plotkin and Orenstein on Vaccines 4th edition. The evidence on benefits and adverse effects is outlined in this publication.

Despite numerous subsequent emails, registered letters, FOI (Freedom of Information) requests and FOI appeals she never budged from her original position that the two textbooks contained the primary references. However, she refused to cite the primary references so that I could examine them.

I subsequently discovered that Dr Darina O'Flanagan was 'just' a medical doctor. She assumed that what she had studied at medical school is correct, in particular the Germ Theory of Disease and the existence of pathogenic viruses. Medical doctors are not the relevant technical experts on viruses, even though they strongly recommend vaccinations, vaccinate us and the vast majority of us defer to their expert opinion.

Over time, I focused my efforts on the virologists because they are the relevant technical experts. The National Virus Reference Laboratory (NVRL) is affiliated with the School of Medicine at University College Dublin. I emailed and wrote registered letters to its then Director Professor Bill Hall PhD MD and a colleague of his Dr Jeff Connell PhD.

I emailed Professor Bill Hall on Friday 5 February 2010 asking him for the scientific proof for the existence of pathogenic viruses. It was a lengthy email requesting scientific papers proving the existence of the measles virus and the bird flu virus—H1N1. Bird Flu was a major topic in 2010 and the great fear then was that there would be a bird flu pandemic, of a scale similar to the Spanish Flu. I have reproduced the last few paragraph of this email:

> Professor Hall I accept that it is your opinion and that of your colleagues that pathogenic viruses such as H1N1 and measles exist. What I am interested is the primary evidence on which any expert such as you should base his opinion.
>
> If this primary evidence is readily available, as it should be, if the case for the existence of these pathogenic viruses is so self-evident, it should be possible for you Professor Bill Hall to provide me and more importantly Dr Stefan Lanka with the relevant scientific publications. If you cannot do so, then you must publicly state why this is not possible.

> Why do we vaccinate against viruses that we cannot prove to exist, even though it is technically possible to isolate real viruses (which are harmless) and it would be also possible to isolate allegedly pathogenic viruses if they actually existed?
>
> Professor Bill Hall, you as Director of the NVRL and as the Irish expert on so-called pathogenic viruses know full well that the techniques used by your organisation to identify viruses are indirect methods which assume that these viruses actually exist. It has been possible since the early 1970s to biochemically characterise viruses. It has been possible since the early 1930s to photograph pathogenic viruses, if they existed, with an electron microscope. It is now possible to directly prove the existence of these viruses.
>
> Professor Hall I believe that you can become a great scientist and more importantly a truly great human being. You have the ability to expose the criminal lie that pathogenic viruses exist. This is a great responsibility. The truth will be eventually revealed but you have the tremendous opportunity to greatly shorten the timescale.
>
> Please do the right thing.

I got no response.

Over a year later, on Thursday 19 May 2011, I e-mailed Professor Bill Hall and positively asserted that pathogenic viruses cannot exist and requested him to refute me.

> Dear Professor Hall,
>
> I assert that there is no scientific evidence for the existence of the mumps and H1N1 viruses (as two examples of allegedly pathogenic viruses) because these viruses have not been:-

> 1 isolated from the host cell;
>
> 2 biochemically characterised; and
>
> 3 photographed.
>
> The National Virus Reference Laboratory use indirect techniques for virus detection such as PCR, which are meaningless, because these 'viruses' have never been directly proven to exist in the first place.
>
> I have repeatedly asked you for scientific papers proving the existence of these allegedly pathogenic viruses, as well as other viruses such as measles and H5N1. In your capacity as Director of the National Virus Reference Laboratory, and therefore as the most eminent authority in Ireland on pathogenic viruses, it is vitally important that you either concur with or refute my assertion that these viruses do not exist.
>
> Given that the Ectocarpus siliculosus virus with a diameter of approximately 120nm has been already isolated, there is no reason why all other pathogenic viruses of a similar diameter from 60 nm to 180nm (according to Dr Stefan Lanka) cannot be isolated in a similar manner.
>
> If you do not rebut my assertion that these viruses do not exist, and produce scientific evidence for your opinion within the next 21 days, then I will take it that you agree that there is no scientific evidence for the existence of any pathogenic virus.
>
> The Germ Theory of Disease is wrong and pathogenic viruses do not exist.

The reason why I positively asserted that they could not exist was in the forlorn hope that he would feel obliged to reply and deny my assertion. However, he ignored me.

What is the Diameter of Pathogenic Viruses?

For the first five years of my correspondence with the health authorities, I repeatedly asked them to cite the scientific paper, which proves the existence of a pathogenic virus and demonstrates how the virus has been:

1. Isolated;
2. Biochemically Characterised; and
3. Photographed.

I decided to change my question to the virologists and assume that they are correct and that viruses exist. I distilled my query to a two-part question: What are the diameters of pathogenic viruses and how did you measure them?

On Monday 18 July 2011, I emailed the NVRL in response to a letter I had received a few days earlier from the then Minister for Health Dr James Reilly MD.

> Dear Professor Bill Hall & Dr Jeff Connell,
>
> Please find below the response to my letter from the Minister for Health concerning proof for the existence of the H1NI virus and the mumps virus.
>
> The Minister writes:-
>
> *The role of the Irish Health Service is not to disprove the basic fundamental research but to confirm the presence or absence of the virus for individual patients.*
>
> As senior employees of the National Virus Reference Laboratory, you both know that the techniques you use for detecting so-called pathogenic viruses are indirect techniques, which are based on the assumption that the

> Germ Theory of Disease is correct and that pathogenic viruses exist.
>
> Again, I ask, what is the diameter of the H1N1 virus and the mumps virus? Why can you not isolate these alleged viruses in the same manner that Dr Stefan Lanka isolated the Ectocarpus silculosus virus, which has a diameter of 120nm?
>
> The truth will out eventually as has recently happened with the phone-hacking practices of the Murdock empire and also with the clerical sexual abuse scandals.
>
> I hope and pray that both of you will facilitate the truth emerging to the general public that pathogenic viruses cannot be isolated, because they do not exist!

I got no response.

***

I emailed Professor Bill Hall about a meeting of the Global Virus Network (GVN) at University College Dublin, which he had organised for mid-October 2011.

> Dear Professor Hall,
>
> Could your colleagues at the Global Virus Network provide me with the diameters of all known pathogenic viruses and explain to Dr Stefan Lanka how you isolated and measured them?
>
> As you know, I have repeatedly asked you for this information. If these viruses exist, why can you not provide it? Logic tells me why, but what about you?

I got no response.

The Global Virus Network (GVN) has people such as Bob Gallo (co-discoverer of the alleged HIV-virus), Dr Reinhard Kurth from Germany and of course Professor Bill Hall. It had its inaugural meeting in March 2011 in Washington DC. The program for the weekend meeting in October 2011 in Dublin included "Discussion on the most significant viral threats as agreed by GVN members." This all looks reasonable and even laudable on the surface. However, there is a major problem—there should be no viral threat because pathogenic viruses cannot exist, because no one has ever seen or purified them.

The key players involved in the Global Virus Network know about Dr Stefan Lanka's work. They all know that there is no evidence for the existence of pathogenic viruses. At this stage, the only possible interpretation one can construct for the Global Virus Network is that it is all about creating a manufactured event (a global swine-flu / bird-flu pandemic, or as it turned out in 2020, a coronavirus pandemic) which will have to be treated by vaccines. The vaccine will cause the real pandemic, which is what happened with the Spanish Flu.

***

I had been in an admittedly one-way correspondence with Professor Bill Hall about the existence of all pathogenic viruses for several years because he never responded to any of my many e-mails. I even sent him registered letters in the forlorn hope that he would feel obliged to respond.

In October 2011, I discovered that UCD and the National Virus Reference Laboratory (NVRL) were subject to Freedom of Information (FOI). I made an FOI request to UCD (foi@ucd.ie) on Wednesday 5 October 2011 requesting the diameters of all known pathogenic viruses. Over two months later on 19 December 2011, I received a letter from Mary Hogan, University Records Manager at UCD. The relevant extract is shown:

> . . . Having considered the provision of the Acts, I have decided to refuse to grant access to the requested records. The National Virus Reference Laboratory has, as stated in your request, "the technical ability to detect pathogenic viruses". However, the records you request are not held. I must therefore invoke Section 10(1) (a) of the Acts, which states:
>
> "10(1) A head to whom a request under section 7 is made may refuse to grant the request if the record concerned does not exist or cannot be found after all reasonable steps to ascertain its whereabouts have been taken."

I was busy getting ready for Christmas and spent some time thinking about this FOI response, which I found to be extremely interesting. Professor Bill Hall did not lie. He did not make up diameters for pathogenic viruses, which he could have. However, his reply was ambiguous. Could I get him to admit that pathogenic viruses had never been purified?

I thought a lot about all this a lot over the Christmas holidays. I was getting tired of all this one-way correspondence. I had run out of energy and enthusiasm for this endeavour. I wanted definitive answers from the NVRL. I had to get my FOI appeal as accurate and as specific as possible. I prayed a lot about it and asked the Holy Spirit for guidance in drafting my appeal.

Dear Professor Bill Hall PhD MD,

I am appealing your denial of my FOI request. I requested from you, (in your position as Director of the National Virus Reference Laboratory—NVRL), the diameters of all known pathogenic viruses. You denied my FOI request because the "records . . . are not held". I am appealing this because your response is ambiguous.

Does your response mean that the records do not exist because no pathogenic virus has ever been isolated? Or, do you mean that pathogenic viruses have been isolated, but their diameters have never been measured? I want to know precisely what you mean by your FOI response that the records I requested "are not held".

Isolation of pathogenic viruses

If you state in your response to my FOI appeal that pathogenic viruses have been isolated, I would like you to provide me with the scientific publications demonstrating this:

Virus	**Scientific Publication**
Mumps Measles H1N1 H5N1 etc	Scientific publication proving the existence of the respective virus and stating how it was isolated biochemically characterized and photographed.

I have been asking you for this information for over three years, but have never received a response.

No pathogenic virus has ever been isolated

I am in a surreal position because of my original FOI request. I made it knowing that no such record can exist, because these pathogenic viruses have never been isolated in the first place. I would like the NVRL to confirm in my FOI appeal what Dr Stefan Lanka has been stating for years, which is that no pathogenic virus has ever been:

1) Isolated;

2) Its diameter measured;

3) Its viral coat and core biochemically characterised; and

4) Photographed.

Koch's Postulates

Robert Koch (1843–1910) came up with four postulates that must be satisfied in order to prove the existence of a pathogenic virus. The first postulate states that the virus must be observable in a tissue sample of a person infected with the virus. The second postulate states that the pathogenic virus must be capable of being isolated from the tissue sample.

Therefore, according to Koch's postulates, pathogenic viruses cannot be claimed to exist because they have never been isolated.

Marine Brown Alga Ectocarpus siliculosus Virus

Dr Stefan Lanka succeeded in isolating the Marine Brown Alga Ectocarpus silculosus virus. Its diameter is 120 nm. He also biochemically characterized the viral coat and core and photographed it. This virus did not cause its host to become diseased, but rather the Marine Brown Alga Ectocarpus silculosus thrived in its presence.

In one litre of seawater, there are millions of viruses, but they are not pathogenic. These non-pathogenic viruses can be isolated, measured, photographed and biochemically characterised. Would it be possible for Professor Bill Hall to confirm that these non-pathogenic viruses do exist?

Having discovered a non-pathogenic virus, Dr Lanka was deemed to be an expert on all viruses including pathogenic viruses. He initially examined the scientific literature on the HIV-virus. To his surprise he could not discover any scientific paper where a scientist claims to have isolated the HIV-virus. He also examined the scientific literature concerning viruses that we vaccinate our children against, and discovered that there were no scientific papers demonstrating the isolation of the mumps, measles, rubella viruses etc.

Professor Hall, does it not concern you that it is possible to isolate non-pathogenic viruses with diameters of 120nm and less, but it is impossible to isolate any pathogenic virus?

Measles virus

The first of Koch's postulates is apparently satisfied because one can observe what appears to be the "measles virus' in a tissue sample taken from a child with measles.

Professor Antoine Béchamp (1816–1908) came up with the idea of pleomorphism, which is that cells change shape in response to disease conditions.

The question is do the cells change shape because of an external pathogenic virus—the measles virus—or do they change shape in response to disease conditions; in response to the child having measles? Is measles internally generated? Or is it caused by an external agent—the measles virus?

Given that, no one has ever isolated the measles virus: One must logically conclude that the reason is that it does not exist. Dr Stefan Lanka is so confident about this he is offering €100,000 to any scientist who isolates the measles virus and states its diameter.

Dr Stefan Lanka further elaborates that pathogenic viruses do not exist in humans, animals or plants.

FOI Appeal Summary

In order to be able to measure the diameter of a pathogenic virus, one would have to isolate it first. I take it that this is self-evident.

I want Professor Bill Hall to address the following three issues so that his response to my FOI appeal is unambiguous. I want Professor Bill Hall to confirm that to his current knowledge:

1) There is no record in existence worldwide where a scientist has isolated a pathogenic virus and measured its diameter.

And, to remove any possibility of ambiguity, I want Professor Bill Hall to confirm that to his current knowledge:

2) There is no scientific publication in existence worldwide, where any scientist claims to have isolated any pathogenic virus, let alone measured its diameter, biochemically characterised the coat and the core of the virus, and photographed it.

> 3) Thirdly, I would like Professor Bill Hall to state whether he is concerned by the inability of any scientist (or scientific institution such as WHO, RKI, CDC, NVRL, CRID etc) to isolate any pathogenic virus.
>
> Provided that I get a clear unambiguous response to these three issues, you will be happy to know Professor Bill Hall, that this will finally conclude my correspondence with you.

I receive a response from John Coman, Corporate and Legal Affairs Secretary at University College Dublin on Monday 6 February 2012; it was more or less a re-statement of their response to my first FOI appeal. The pertinent extract is shown:

> I have now reviewed your original request and Ms Hogan's response to it and wish to inform you that I am upholding Ms Hogan's decision.
>
> I have now considered the additional questions raised in your request for internal review, as summarised in the final paragraph "FOI Appeal Summary". The points in relation to which confirmation is requested, refer to matters of academic research and cannot be dealt with under Freedom of Information Acts. The University is committed to its obligations under the Act to provide requesters with access to records held by it and with reasons for its decision that affect them. In this case, we regret that we cannot assist you further.
>
> Under the Acts, the university is required to advise you of your right, following receipt of your internal review decision, to make a further review application by writing to the Information Commissioner, 18 Lower Leeson Street, Dublin 2.

On Friday 24 February 2012, having received the minimalist response to my second FOI appeal from University College Dublin, I emailed the Office of the Information Commissioner (OIC). I included the FOI response from Professor Bill Hall at UCD NVRL and the response from Dr Darina O'Flanagan (the Director of the HPSC), which I believe are contradictory. The relevant extract from my email to the OIC follows:

> Please find attached the decision on my FOI appeal from the NVRL. You will note that the NVRL is reiterating that the "record does not exist". This is in contrast with the decision made by the HPSC, which is that the "record does exist". These two FOI responses are clearly contradictory.
>
> You will note that both the NVRL and the HPSC are being minimalistic in their FOI responses. They cannot state the diameters of any pathogenic viruses. They cannot cite any scientific papers, where any scientist has managed to isolate any pathogenic virus. They cannot do any of this because pathogenic viruses do not exist, but they cannot admit that.
>
> The key point is that if pathogenic viruses existed they should be able to state their respective diameters. They can't and this has been proven by their two FOI responses.
>
> It is clear that these issues are more than just "matters of academic research", because I am questioning the existence of pathogenic viruses.
>
> My assertion that pathogenic viruses do not exist has major implications:

1) It means that at the very least the Irish state is wasting a colossal amount of tax-payers money on vaccines against phantom viruses; and

2) There is the most significant issue of the damage caused to Irish children by vaccines, such as the recent narcolepsy cases afflicting 40 Irish children because of the swine-flu vaccine.

I appreciate any help you can give me in this regard.

I had a series of emails and phone calls with Anne Harwood from the Office of the Information Commissioner. Her response on Friday 24 February 2012: "They are two separate decisions from two separate public bodies and have to be treated separately for the purposes of any review to the Information Commissioner."

Anne phoned me and explained again how the FOI legislation worked and that any appeal would have to be on an individual basis and would be on purely procedural FOI legislation and not on the substantive issue concerning the existence of pathogenic viruses. For this reason, I did not make an appeal to the Office of the Information Commissioner about the contradictory FOI responses from two different government bodies.

***

As I live in Northern Ireland, I decided in February 2012 to ask the authorities in London (Health Protection Agency—HPA, foi@hpa.org.uk) about the diameters of viruses. In March 2012, I got a detailed response from Leigh Hopkins, a Freedom of Information Officer. She confirmed that they held some of the information I required. She provided some interesting background notes on the size of viruses:

> Virus dimensions are often quoted as a diameter, however, this terminology can be quite misleading as it suggests that they are circular or spherical. The electron microscope allows us to see that while this is true for some viruses, for others it is not. For example, the smallest types of virus known to infect man are the parvoviruses (a parvovirus is the causative agent of "slapped-cheek" in children) which are roughly spherical particles with diameters of about 20nm. The largest viruses are the pox viruses (causative agents of smallpox and molluscum contagiosum) which are not spherical but brick-shaped or oval and are approximately 200nm by 400nm. The most extreme deviation from the spherical shape are the filoviruses (the most infamous type being the ebola virus), which are seen as filaments ("filo" comes from the latin word for filament) about 80nm wide and many hundreds (occasionally even thousands) of nm in length.

I was surprised. She stated the diameters of various viruses. Her response was much better than what I had obtained from the Irish authorities. Any ordinary person with no training in virology would say—well that is it then and just leave it. However, that was not it. Presumably, they must have purified the virus first, before they measured its diameter.

> First of all, thank you for your help. I appreciate the efforts you went to in obtaining this information.
>
> I have now considered your response in detail. You have answered my FOI request for the diameters of pathogenic viruses. Thank you!

> I wish to make a further FOI request, which is I would like the name of the scientific publication which proves the existence of a particular pathogenic virus.
>
> I understand that the measles virus has a diameter of 150nm according to the spreadsheet that was attached. My FOI request, using the measles virus as an example is can you please cite the scientific publication where a scientist has isolated the measles virus and measured its diameter and obtained a measurement of approximately 150nm?
>
> Thanks for your help in this matter. I really appreciate it.

She replied, and told me that the Health Protection Agency "does not hold the information I have requested". I replied almost immediately.

> You gave me some references in a previous e-mail, which state that the measles virus has a diameter of 150nm. My question is: How do you know? Presumably, the scientists must have isolated the virus first prior to its diameter being measured?
>
> In your response, you state: "Other than publicly available information, for example, peer reviewed journals and reference books the HPA does not hold the information specified in your question".
>
> All I ask is that you cite a scientific paper, (held outside the HPA), where some scientist has managed to isolate the measles virus and measure its diameter and come up with a diameter of 150nm?
>
> I appreciate your help.

On Thursday 5 April 2012, I received the following response from another HPA employee called Gloria Akinyemi.

> Thank you for your email dated 29 March. Regarding your further question regarding a scientific paper on measles virus size please see the below information.
>
> Waterson, A.P., Cruickshank, J.G., Laurence, G.D., and Kanarek, A.D. (1961). The nature of the Measles virus. Virology 15;379-382.
>
> This paper appears to be generally credited with being the first to show the fine structure of the agent responsible for causing measles. They describe irregularly shaped (ie pleimorphic) virions that "were approximately circular or oval in outline" and with an overall diameter of 120-250nm.
>
> I hope you have found this information helpful.

Success! This paper is not freely available on the internet and you have to pay to access it. I forwarded the e-mail to Dr Stefan Lanka and asked him for a comment. He replied a week later that the paper showed "cellular particles and debris". In other words, the paper had not demonstrated how they purified the measles virus. How were they able to measure a diameter between 120nm–250nm, if they could not purify it first?

I emailed Gloria on 25 April 2012 and asked, "Do the HPA (or other UK authorities) confirm the presence of the measles virus by isolating it? If so, may I have a paper describing how they isolate the measles virus?" She replied on 8 May 2012 with what I thought was a good detailed response:

> We don't confirm the presence of the measles virus by isolating it, we confirm the disease has been detected by two different methods: 1. detecting an IgM antibody response

> to the virus in a patient's blood sample, 2. Detecting the virus itself using a molecular test called the polymerase chain reaction (PCR). The virus can be isolated in tissue culture, but this is not used for diagnosis.

I immediately replied to her:

> Thanks for that. Will you provide me with a recent scientific paper demonstrating how the measles virus was isolated, and its diameter measured? My presumption is that the virus must be isolated first before its diameter can be measured?
>
> I am sorry to be so persistent, but I want a recent scientific paper, which demonstrates how the measles virus was isolated using modern technology.

Gloria replied promptly, two days later on Thursday 10 May 2012.

> Thank you for your below email dated 8 May.
>
> However, we have provided you with information regarding papers you can refer to regarding the measurements of measles virus size. This was sent to you on 5th April. We are unable to provide you with this paper due to publishing rights not being owned by the HPA. However, this information is in the public domain if you choose to locate it.
>
> We have also confirmed the HPA does not confirm the presence of the measles virus by isolating it, we confirm the disease has been detected by two different methods: 1. detecting an IgM antibody response to the virus in a patients blood sample, 2. Detecting the virus itself using a molecular test called the polymerase chain reaction

> (PCR). The virus can be isolated in tissue culture, but this is not used for diagnosis.
>
> In your request of 8 May, you are now requesting information that confirms your opinion, and are choosing not to acknowledge the scientific information that has been provided to you by the HPA.
>
> We have provided you with our response to your questions regarding measles and have no further information to add to our reply. I apologise if you remain unsatisfied with the information you have received, and suggest you may wish to contact the Department for Health in relation to virus detection policy issues.

That was the end of our 'conversation'. Nonetheless, I was grateful. The NVRL had simply said that "No Record Exists", and had not elaborated on what they meant despite multiple requests. The English authorities had provided more detail and explained that they use indirect methods: antibody testing and the PCR test. They confirmed what I already knew: No one has ever purified the measles virus.

Density Gradient Centrifugation

I made the following appeal to the Office of the Information Commissioner in Dublin on 27 September 2016 following another case of 'No Record Exists' from the National Virus Reference Laboratory. The pertinent extract is shown:

I have a number of points:

> 1) Dr Darina O'Flanagan from the HPSC (darina.oflanagan@hpsc.ie) stated under FOI that a medical text-book contained the primary references, i.e. primary scientific papers, which proved the existence of the mumps, measles

and rubella viruses, by demonstrating how they were isolated or purified. However, she repeatedly refused to provide me with the primary references. Her FOI response directly contradicts the responses from the NVRL, which are that 'no record exists' in relation to the isolation of any pathogenic virus. She should either cite one reference for the measles virus for example; or admit like that NVRL has, that 'no record exists', and retract her previous FOI response.

2) The NVRL has correctly stated that no scientific publication exists, in which a scientist has managed to isolate any alleged pathogenic virus (such as mumps, measles, rubella, H1N1, HIV, H1N1 etc). 'No Record Exists' is their response, and I agree with it. It is not possible to isolate any pathogenic virus because they do not exist.

3) I understand the 'density centrifugation technique' is the standard textbook technique for isolating viruses. The NVRL have stated under FOI that they do not use this technique to isolate pathogenic viruses.

4) If pathogenic viruses existed, it should be possible to isolate them. This is also the second Koch postulate: *The microorganism must be isolated from a diseased organism and grown in pure culture.* The scientists observe what they believe to be the mumps, measles and rubella viruses in a blood sample (Koch's first postulate), but they cannot isolate any of these alleged pathogenic viruses.

5) I accept that the vast majority of scientists and medical doctors worldwide believe in the existence of pathogenic viruses. However, a belief is not enough; it must be supported by physical evidence and of this I have seen none. I have not seen the scientific paper, which demonstrates how any pathogenic virus was isolated.

6) Dr Stefan Lanka PhD isolated the Marine Brown Algae Ectocarpus Siliculosus virus, which exists in sea-water and is non-pathogenic. It has a diameter of 120nm. In one litre of sea-water there are thousands of these non-pathogenic viruses and they can be isolated—they do exist! Again, I have asked the NVRL if they agree that this virus and others have been isolated but they have refused to comment. It is possible to isolate non-pathogenic viruses, but somehow it is not possible to isolate any pathogenic viruses?

7) Dr Stefan Lanka states that currently almost 300 non-pathogenic viruses have already been proven to exist, because they have been isolated, biochemically characterised and photographed. Furthermore, their diameter has been accurately measured. Again, do the NVRL agree with this? They have not responded to my repeated queries about this. The issue here is: If it is possible to isolate non-pathogenic viruses, why is it impossible to isolate pathogenic viruses.

8) In summary, the NVRL are correct when the say that 'no record exists' in relation to the isolation of any pathogenic virus. However, my question is why does 'no record exist'. If pathogenic viruses existed, it should be possible to isolate them, and there should be a record. The NVRL are being minimalist in their vacuous response that 'no record exists'.

9) The broader picture behind this is that the 'Germ Theory of Disease' is wrong. The Achilles' Heel of modern medicine and biology, which refutes this erroneous belief in the Germ Theory of Disease is that pathogenic viruses do not exist. They do not exist because they cannot be isolated. There are alternative explanations behind what they currently believe to be the measles virus, which is

explained by the work of Dr Stefan Lanka and Dr Ryke Geerd Hamer.

10) It is impossible to prove a negative. I cannot prove that pathogenic viruses do not exist. If someone claims that there is a man on the moon, it is their responsibility to provide the evidence, which supports this assertion. It is not my responsibility to prove them wrong. Similarly, the NVRL (National Virus Reference Laboratory) claim that pathogenic viruses exist. However, they cannot provide any evidence, which supports this assertion. They cannot isolate any pathogenic virus—No Record Exists is the standard response.

I believe I have provided the key points supporting my appeal against the NVRL decision. I want them to explain why it is impossible to isolate any pathogenic virus. I want them to explain why 'no record exists'.

I welcome any queries from your investigator

A Senior Investigator with the OIC, Stephen Rafferty, wrote a detailed report dated 17 January 2017 about his findings.

Case Number:	160377
Applicant:	Mr James McCumiskey.
FOI Body:	University College Dublin (UCD)
Issue:	Whether UCD was justified in refusing to release records relating to whether the National Virus Reference Laboratory (NVRL) had ever applied a density gradient centrifugation technique to isolate pathogenic viruses on the ground that it holds no such records.

Review:	Conducted in accordance with section 22(2) of the FOI Act by Stephen Rafferty, Senior Investigator, who is authorised by the Information Commissioner to conduct this review
Decision:	The Senior Investigator affirmed the decision of UCD
Right of Appeal:	Section 24 of the FOI Act sets out detailed provisions for an appeal to the High Court by a party to a review, or any other person affected by the decision. In summary, such an appeal, normally on a point of law, must be initiated not later than four weeks after notice of the decision was given to the person bringing the appeal.

Background

According to its website, the UCD NVRL provides a diagnostic and reference service for clinicians investigating viral infections throughout Ireland. The laboratory is affiliated to the UCD School of Medicine. By email dated 27 May 2016, the applicant referenced an article by Dr Stefan Lanka and asked the NVRL to confirm under FOI "whether the NVRL have ever applied this density gradient centrifugation technique to attempt to isolate any so-called pathogenic virus? And if so what was the outcome?" In its decision of 27 June 2016, UCD stated that, in so far as the request can be interpreted as a valid request for records held by it, no records are held which would provide an answer or the confirmation sought.

The applicant sought an internal review of that decision and on 14 September 2016, UCD affirmed its original decision to refuse the request on the ground that it holds no records that would provide an answer to the applicant's query and the density gradient centrifugation technique is not used at the NVRL. The applicant sought a review by this Office of UCD's decision on 23 September 2016.

Scope of Review

The scope of this review is solely concerned with whether UCD was justified in refusing the applicant's request under section 15(10(a) of the FOI Act on the ground that it holds no relevant records.

Preliminary Matters

It seems to me that the applicant did not fully understand the nature of the rights afforded by the FOI Act when he submitted his FOI request to UCD. The Act provides for a right of access to records held by FOI bodies. This means that if the information sought is not contained in a record held by the FOI body then the body cannot grant the request. The Act does not require FOI bodies to answer questions or to create records, which do not exist. Where a request is made in the form of a request for specific information as opposed to a request for specific records, as was the case with the applicant's request, this Office takes the view that such requests should be treated as requests for relevant records that exist as of the date of the request that contain the information sought. In this case, UCD correctly considered the applicant's request as a request for records, which indicate whether the NVRL have ever applied the density gradient centrifugation technique "to attempt to isolate any so-called pathogenic virus".

It is also important to note that UCD is responsible for considering only those records that it holds or that are under its control. It appears that the applicant interpreted

UCD's decision as a statement that no record exists anywhere. I note, for example, that in his application to this Office, he argued that the NVRL had stated that "no record exists in the world". This is an incorrect interpretation of UCD's decision. Rather, UCD stated that it held no records that contain the information he was seeking.

Analysis and Findings

Section 15(1)(a) provides that an FOI body may refuse to grant a request where the records sought do not exist or cannot be found after all reasonable steps to ascertain their whereabouts have been taken. The role of this Office in such cases is to review the decision of the body and to decide whether that decision was justified. This means that I must have regard to the evidence available to the decision maker and the reasoning used by the decision maker in arriving at his/her decision and also must assess the adequacy of the searches conducted by the FOI body in looking for relevant records. The evidence in "search" cases consists of the steps actually taken to search for records, along with miscellaneous other evidence about the record management practices of the FOI body, on the basis of which the FOI body concluded that the steps taken to search for records were reasonable. On the basis of the information provided, this Office forms a view as to whether the decision maker was justified in coming to the decision that the records sought do not exist or cannot be found.

In its submission to this Office, UCD stated that this was not a case which was based on search details, or its record-keeping practices. According to UCD, the NVRL Laboratory Director stated that the density-gradient technique is not used by the NVRL as it is "an old method" which has been "superseded by more modern

> techniques". UCD stated that the techniques used by the NVRL were in accordance with international best practice. Furthermore, UCD stated that the NVRL has never used density gradient centrifugation to isolate viruses. It stated that consequently, it holds no records containing the information sought by the applicant. I have no reason to doubt that this is the case.
>
> Indeed, it seems to me that the applicant did not expect UCD to hold relevant records. In his application for internal review, he argued that pathogenic viruses do not exist, that the density gradient centrifugation technique will be unable to isolate any "alleged pathogenic virus", and that UCD's response confirmed what he already knew. He stated that he wished to ascertain from the NVRL why it is "impossible to isolate any so-called pathogenic virus". It seems to me that the applicant's request, as set out in that email, was based on a misunderstanding of the nature of the access rights afforded by the FOI Act and of the requirements imposed on bodies such as UCD to process requests for access to records they hold.
>
> Having taken all of the above into account, I am of the view that UCD was justified in refusing the applicant's request under section 15(1) (a) on the ground that it does not hold the records sought.
>
> **Decision**
>
> Having carried out a review under section 22(2) of the Freedom of Information Act 2014, I hereby affirm UCD's decision to refuse the applicant's request on the ground that no relevant records exist.

I was happy with the findings in the report, particularly the admission by the NVRL Laboratory Director that the density-gradient technique is an "old method", which has been "superseded by more modern techniques". The NVRL also admitted the technique they used were in accordance with international best practice and that they had never used density gradient centrifugation to purify viruses. I believe that these admissions would be useful in a future court case. In addition, I believe that the NVRL had confirmed that they are not operating in a scientific manner. Why would the NVRL not try to purify a pathogenic virus using Density Gradient Centrifugation? Why would they not carry out this simple control experiment?

Although I was happy that the investigator had gotten some useful information from the National Virus Reference Laboratory, I was unhappy that he had taken such a purist view of 'No Record Exists'. I had a number of conversations with OIC employees and they explained their position to me. They were taking a literal view and they repeatedly emphasised that I agree with the NVRL that no record exists. Therefore, if no record exists, the NVRL are not obliged to provide the record. However, the real issue though is why no record exists. Could it be that viruses do not exist and that this is the reason why no record exists? The OIC were unwilling to challenge the science, but I was grateful that they explained their opinion to me and that the FOI route could not provide me with the explicit response I wanted from the NVRL.

Control Experiment to Purify the Measles Virus

I emailed the NVRL on Wednesday 7 March 2018 and asked them to carry out a scientific control experiment using density gradient centrifugation to purify a 'giant virus' and to contrast that with an attempt to purify the measles virus.

FOI Request / Experiment to prove the existence of the measles virus

Dr Lanka states that the scientifically valid method for the isolation of any alleged virus is the density gradient centrifugation technique. This technique is apparently referenced in all current textbooks but for some reason is never used by the laboratories such as the NVRL.

I would like the NVRL to carry out a simple experiment:

1) Attempt to isolate the measles virus using the density gradient centrifugation technique.

2) As a control experiment isolate any so-called giant virus such as the Marine Brown Alga *ectocarpus siliculosus* virus using the density gradient centrifugation technique.

I am certain that it will be impossible to isolate the measles virus or any other alleged pathogenic virus (such as HIV, HPV, H5N1, mumps, rubella, IAVs, novel corona virus etc) because they do not exist. However, it is possible to isolate the so-called giant viruses with a diameter of 120-150nm; I believe almost 3,000 of these giant viruses have to date been isolated by the density gradient centrifugation technique.

A scientist must question all his assumptions and beliefs otherwise the status quo would never change; this is the scientific method; this is real science. I request that the NVRL carry out this simple experiment (and create a new record / scientific paper). I understand from Dr Stefan Lanka that any first year university biology student would be able to carry out this proposed experiment, which is

> simple, cheap and fast to execute. I would like the NVRL to explain the outcome of this experiment.
>
> I believe that the only logical conclusion from this experiment will be the determination that all alleged pathogenic viruses such as for example the mumps, measles and rubella do not exist.
>
> Prove my hypothesis wrong! Create the record, perform the experiment and attempt to isolate the measles virus using the density gradient centrifugation technique.

Debbie Scanlan replied on Friday 23 March 2018 and stated that my request is "not for records held by the University and as such is invalid in terms of Section 11 of the Act". In other words, I am asking them to create a record, perform a scientific experiment, which they refuse to do. I asked the NVRL to move beyond the legalities of the FOI Act, carry out the control experiment and create the record. Instead, they hide behind the legalities of the FOI Act, which only requires them to provide access to records they hold. The NVRL is not acting in a scientific manner; it is not a scientific institution.

Having had no response to my original request to create the record, on Thursday 14 June 2018, I emailed the NVRL once again:

> Did the NVRL attempt to purify the measles virus using the density centrifugation technique? If not why not? Or alternatively, can you cite any record / scientific publication where the measles virus has been purified? If you state that "no record exists", can you explain why it is impossible to purify the measles virus? Can you explain why we vaccinate our children against a phantom virus? I am not interested in current scientific consensus. I am

> looking for the evidence or the record underlying your belief in the existence of the measles virus—Please provide it.

They were unwilling to carry out the control experiment and create the record.

***

On 19 June 2018, I received the following response from Public Health England to my request for them to carry out a similar control experiment.

> Re: measles
>
> Thank you for your request for information addressed to Public Health England (PHE). In accordance with Section 1(1)(a) of the Freedom of Information Act 2000 (the Act) I can confirm that PHE does not hold the information you have specified.
>
> You asked:
>
> *FOI Request / Experiment to prove the existence of the measles virus*
>
> *Dr Stefan Lanka states that the scientifically valid method for the isolation of any alleged virus is the density gradient centrifugation technique. This technique is apparently referenced in all current microbiology textbooks but for some reason is never used by the laboratories such as the VRD.*
>
> *I would like the VRD to carry out a simple experiment:*
>
> *1) Attempt to isolate the measles virus using the density gradient centrifugation technique; and*

> *2) As a control experiment isolate any so-called giant virus such as the Marine Brown Alga ectocarpus siliculosus virus using the density gradient centrifugation technique.*
>
> *I hypothesise that it will be impossible to isolate the measles virus or any other alleged pathogenic virus (such as HIV, HPV, H5N1, mumps, rubella etc) because they do not exist. However, it is possible to isolate the so-called giant viruses with a diameter of 120-150nm; I believe almost 3,000 of these giant viruses have to date been isolated by the density gradient centrifugation technique. These viruses, which have been proven to exist, are non-pathogenic and in fact are beneficial for the host.*
>
> Your request for information is not a valid FOI request. https://ico.org.uk/for-organisations/guide-to-freedom-of-information/receiving-a-request/
>
> Furthermore, PHE is not obliged to create new information to respond to a request under the FOI Act.

Just like the National Virus Reference Laboratory in Dublin, Public Health England will not carry out a scientific experiment and create a record. They too hide behind the legalities of FOI legislation.

Freedom of Information

There is no Freedom of Information. There is management of information. Freedom of Information is a misnomer. Information that is inconvenient or embarrassing to the information owner will not be released.

The FOI Officers in England were initially more helpful than their counterparts were in Ireland. However, when it came down to citing a scientific publication where the measles virus was purified, they were unable and the correspondence was cut off.

They were also unwilling to enter into dialogue, carry out the scientific experiment I suggested and attempt to purify a pathogenic virus and create a new record.

I never appealed the 'No Record Exists' to the Information Commissioner in England because I had already made the appeal to the Information Commissioner in Ireland. I found that process useful, because the investigator was able to glean useful information from the National Virus Reference Laboratory, such as the fact they consider density gradient centrifugation an "old method" for the identification of viruses. This is a significant point because it is the standard method used to purify bionts—bacteriophages and so-called 'giant viruses'.

I had gone as far as I could with Freedom of Information. No virologist has ever purified any pathogenic virus: No Record Exists.

Chapter 7

The Corona Reset

An Unnecessary Crisis

The Corona Crisis should have never happened.

If the scientists and doctors had heeded Professor Béchamp rather than Louis Pasteur, the Germ Theory of Disease would never have been established. If the scientists and doctors had heeded Robert Remak rather than Rudolph Virchow, we would not have had cellular pathology and all its supporting dogmas. Instead, we would have learned much earlier the importance of the embryonic germ layers with regard to the classification and understanding of all cancers and diseases.

If the medical profession had been willing to test and confirm Dr Ryke Geerd Hamer's Five Biological Laws in the 1980s, this crisis would never have occurred. Dr Hamer suspected that viruses did not exist, and in his writings repeatedly wrote "viruses, if they exist".

Dr Stefan Lanka discovered what he originally called a giant virus in the late 1980s. He subsequently discovered that there is no evidence for the existence of any alleged pathogenic virus. He told his professional colleagues, gave public lectures and helped instigate 'citizen enquiry' in 2000, where ordinary people queried the scientific authorities for proof for the existence of any alleged pathogenic virus. If the virologists at the Robert Koch Institute had responded appropriately to the enquiries of ordinary citizens, they would have finally admitted that pathogenic viruses do not exist.

The German courts confirmed in 2016 that none of the six scientific papers presented proves the existence of the measles virus. Again, if the courts had acted upon this knowledge and had implemented legal changes in accordance with the fact that the measles virus does not exist, the Corona Crisis would have never happened.

If only we had acted rationally, logically and in accordance with the rules of science, we would not be in our current predicament.

The Origin of the Corona Crisis—The Death of Li Wenliang

On 30 December 2019, the ophthalmologist (eye doctor) Li Wenliang in Wuhan wrote a private post to some of his fellow doctors. He warned about an illness that resembled severe acute respiratory syndrome (SARS) at his hospital.

The World Health Organisation stated in April 2003 that the coronavirus was responsible for the outbreak of SARS in Asia. Consequently, Li Wenliang and his fellow medical colleagues great fear was that there would be another SARS outbreak caused by a coronavirus.

One of the recipients of his private text published a screenshot of it on the internet on December 31 2019, and it went 'viral', initially in China and then internationally.

On January 1 2020, the local health authority announced that they had detected 27 cases of viral pneumonia of unknown cause.

On January 3 2020 Li Wenliang along with his medical colleagues were summoned to the Public Security Bureau in Wuhan and made to sign a statement, in which he was accused of spreading rumours—making false statements that disturbed the public order.[19]

On January 8 2020, Li Wenliang treated a patient with glaucoma, who then had a normal body temperature. She developed a fever the next day and a CAT scan showed a lung infection. Two of her relatives also developed a fever. He reported to the hospital that this clearly proved human-human transmission.

Two days later on January 10 2020, he developed a cough, and then a fever the next day. He self-isolated, because he was convinced that his patient had infected him with the SARS-virus.

He was admitted to hospital as a suspected case after a CAT scan showed a lung infection. His parents and some of his colleagues were also admitted.

In a post on Friday 31 January 2020, he wrote that he was in an intensive care unit and had difficulty breathing. The attending doctors carried out countless different tests, which were all negative. After several negative tests, he finally tested positive for the novel coronavirus on Saturday 1 February 2020.

---

19 https://www.thelancet.com/journals/lancet/article/PIIS0140-6736(20)30382-2 Retrieved April 2021

Li Wenliang disseminated his positive test result on the internet with the following words: "Today nucleic acid testing came back with a positive result, the dust has settled, finally diagnosed" (Lanka, 2020:2).

He told a reporter on Wednesday 5 February 2020 that he was still short of breath and his oxygen saturation was very low. Rumours of his death were abroad by 10pm on Thursday 6 February 2020. Mainstream media reported his death on Thursday evening. However, he died in the early hours of Friday February 7 2020.

Li Wenliang is remembered as a whistle-blower, However he was an inadvertent whistle-blower. He was a highly intelligent young doctor, married with one child, and to compound the tragedy his wife was pregnant when he died. His tragic death at such a young age, 33, convinced the Chinese public that a new highly virulent SARS virus was on the rampage, that the authorities were covering up the seriousness of the threat, and that the actual numbers of deaths and casualties were much worse than officially reported. In this context, one can understand the incredible fear and panic that his premature death generated.

SARS—Severe Acute Respiratory Syndrome

SARS is another name for the symptoms of a-typical pneumonia. It was alleged that there was a cluster of patients in Wuhan with a-typical pneumonia. The assumption was that the cause of the a-typical pneumonia was a new variant of the corona virus. They did not investigate other possible causes of a-typical pneumonia such as breathing in poisonous fumes, solvents or other chemical products; the intake of food or liquids can get into the lungs because of difficulties in swallowing and can cause the most severe form of pneumonia—aspiration pneumonia. The doctors were looking for a virus. Consequently, they excluded other possible causes, which prevented the correct handling of the condition (Lanka 2020:2).

Just imagine if all the money spent on dealing with the phantom virus was used to significantly reduce air pollution in Wuhan? This would have materially improved the duration and quality of life for millions of people.

Corona Myths

I want to dispel four high-profile corona myths.

One persistent and colourful myth is that bats caused the corona virus pandemic. Apparently, virologists have known for years that bats have the coronavirus. They have a strong immune system and so they do not succumb to it. Bats and other wild animal were for sale at the Wuhan market. The suspicion is that bats must have infected other animals, who in turn infected humans, and then we had human-human transmission—contagion. The suspicion that bats were the causal factor appears vindicated, because the Chinese authorities subsequently banned the sale of wild animals at the Wuhan market.[20] The World Health Organisation (WHO) also concluded that the coronavirus

20 https://www.thesun.co.uk/news/11669576/wuhan-bans-sale-of-bat-meat-markets-coronavirus/ Retrieved March 2021

was transferred from bats to other animals and then onto humans.[21]

One can easily disprove the myth that bats caused the Corona Crisis. Nobody has ever purified a coronavirus, neither from a bat nor from a human. The novel coronavirus SARS-CoV-2 does not exist. Therefore, the bat theory is another viral myth, as well as a corona myth.

A second corona myth is that the coronavirus originated in a secret Chinese Communist Party government lab and somehow escaped and infected the people of Wuhan. The idea here is that the Chinese were developing a bioweapon, but the experiment failed when the virus escaped.

This myth is easily refutable. First, pathogenic viruses cannot exist in Nature; thus, it is impossible to create a synthetic one.

Second, even if someone has tuberculosis or cholera—there is no human-human transmission, there is no contagion for bacterial diseases. These experiments should be performed in a transparent manner for the public to understand. As mentioned previously, Max von Pettenkofer already proved in 1892 that the ingestion of a large quantity of cholera bacilli does not cause cholera. Cholera bacilli and tubercular bacilli exist, when a person is suffering from cholera or tuberculosis but they are not the cause. A similar experiment was carried out in the US during the Spanish Flu, which proved that contagion did not work for influenza.

---

21 https://uk.news.yahoo.com/coronavirus-bats-wuhan-world-health-organization-112507142.html Retrieved March 2021.

A third corona myth is that of 'shedding'. According to this myth, vaccinated people shed the spike protein or the mRNA (messenger RNA), thereby infecting the unvaccinated and causing them to get ill. Another variant of this myth is that the vaccines supercharge the existing SARS-CoV-2 virus and makes it highly virulent when it sheds. Again, these myths are easily refutable. Viruses do not exist. There is no such thing as contagion or human-human transmission. Thus, vaccinated people do not pose any danger to unvaccinated people. Shedding is fear mongering by people who are justifiably anti-vaccine because of their known toxicity but nonetheless, still believe in the existence of viruses.

The fourth corona myth is that the SARS-CoV-2 vaccines are bioweapons. This myth implies and assumes that normal childhood vaccines are effective but that the SARS-CoV-2 vaccines are particularly toxic. Again, these vaccines may be more toxic than normal childhood vaccines but all vaccines are toxic.

No Record Exists of SARS-CoV-2

I wanted confirmation from the National Virus Reference Laboratory (NVRL) in Dublin that they too had never purified the SARS-CoV-2 virus. After some deliberation, I finally emailed them on Wednesday 19 February 2020 because of the impending corona pandemic. I initially hesitated because I knew they could not tell me anything substantive about the purification of the SARS-CoV-2 virus. Nonetheless, I wanted it on the record that I had enquired about its existence. I wanted them to confirm that No

Record Exists, that there is no record of the purification of the SARS-CoV-2 virus.

Subject: Novel Coronavirus

Dear Directors / Employees of the NVRL,

In May 2017, you kindly provided me with a scientific paper, which allegedly demonstrated the isolation of the Novel Coronavirus:

Isolation of a novel corona virus from a man with pneumonia in Saudi Arabia Ali Moh Zaki Doctor PhD et al New England Journal of Medicine November 8 2012 https://www.nejm.org/doi/full/10.1056/NEJMoa1211721

The last paragraph on page 1818 is revealing: To further characterise the virus approximately 90% of the virus genome sequence was obtained on sequence analysis with the use of the 454 platform.

Thus, the authors have explicitly admitted that they obtained what they believe is 90% of the genome sequence of this alleged virus. I think we can unanimously agree that 90% is not 100% and they explicitly do not claim to have isolated or purified the Novel Coronavirus. They have merely recreated 90% of what they believe is the genome sequence of the alleged Novel Coronavirus. Despite the title of the paper, the Novel Coronavirus was clearly not purified.

David Crowe, a Canadian Biologist, explains how scientists currently detect the Novel Coronavirus:[22]

22 The following information contained in this email to the NVRL came from David Crowe. Corona Virus Panic, http://theinfectiousmyth.com/book/CoronavirusPanic.pdf Retrieved March 2021.

"Scientists are detecting novel RNA in multiple patients with pneumonia-like conditions, and are assuming that the detection of RNA (which is believed to be wrapped in proteins to form an RNA virus, as coronaviruses are believed to be) is equivalent to isolation of the virus."

Indirect tests such as this clearly do not prove the existence of the Novel Coronavirus.

In the following paper, the scientists were honest enough to admit that they did not purify the Novel Coronavirus: "we did not perform tests for detecting infectious virus in blood". Nonetheless, earlier in the paper they repeatedly referred to the 41 cases (out of 59 similar cases), which tested positive for this RNA as:"41 patients . . . confirmed to be infected with 2019-nCoV."

Huang C et al. Clinical features of patients infected with 2019 novel coronavirus in Wuhan, China. Lancet. 2020 Jan 24. https://www.thelancet.com/journals/lancet/article/PIIS0140-6736(20)30183-5/fulltext

In the following paper, the scientists expressly state, "our study does not fulfil Koch's postulates". In other words, the Novel Coronavirus was not purified and was detected by indirect means.

Zhu N et al. A Novel Coronavirus from Patients with Pneumonia in China, 2019. NEngl J Med. 2020 Jan 14. https://www.nejm.org/doi/full/10.1056/NEJMoa2001017

Thus, the three scientific papers cited above do not prove the existence of the Novel Coronavirus.

FOI Request regarding the Novel Coronavirus

1) I am looking for a scientific paper, which demonstrates how the Novel Coronavirus was purified? Surely, if the

> NVRL is able to detect the Novel Coronavirus, it should also be able to demonstrate how it is purified?
>
> 2) I am also requesting how the NVRL would currently detect the Novel Coronavirus? Do you detect RNA (RiboNucleic Acid) in patients with pneumonia and then assume that the presence of RNA is equivalent to the presence of the Novel Coronavirus?
>
> Or, do you use other indirect means for detecting the Novel Coronavirus?

I received an email on Thursday 27 February confirming my FOI request (FOI12_1_544) on 19 February 2020 and that they would make a decision by 18 March 2020. Two months later—after a few reminder emails—I finally received the FOI decision on May 22 2020.

As I expected, they could not provide a record, which demonstrated the purification of the Novel Coronavirus.

> 1. I must advise you that the University do not hold records to answer your request. As such, section 15 (1) (a) of the FOI Act applies, that states: 15. (1) A head to whom an FOI request is made may refuse to grant the request where—(a) the record concerned does not exist or cannot be found after all reasonable steps to ascertain its whereabouts have been taken
>
> 2. The UCD National Virus Reference Laboratory (NVRL) have confirmed that the current assay being used to detect corona virus is the one recommended by the World Health Organisation (WHO), as published in the attached article.

The attached article was the method developed by Professor Christian Drosten et al to 'detect' the Novel Coronavirus.[23] I appealed this decision one week later on Friday May 29 2020.

> I had two queries in relation to my FOI request. The NVRL answered my second query. I wish to have the first query reviewed.
>
> **FOI Query regarding the Novel Coronavirus:** I am looking for a scientific paper, which demonstrates how the Novel Coronavirus was purified? Surely, if the NVRL is able to detect the Novel Coronavirus, it should also be able to demonstrate how it is purified?
>
> :
>
> It is not tenable to lockdown the entire country because the NVRL believe in the existence of the COVID-19 virus: Belief is not a strong enough basis for such a drastic action. In order to prove the existence of the COVID-19 virus, it would have to be purified, photographed, its diameter measured and be biochemically characterised. Surely, it is beyond a matter of "academic debate" for the NVRL that the COVID-19 virus exists because the country is locked down? Therefore, I am asking for the record, which demonstrates how the COVID-19 virus was purified.
>
> I am stating very clearly that all alleged pathogenic viruses such as the mumps virus, the measles virus and the COVID-19 virus do not exist. If they did exist, it would be possible to purify them.

23 https://pubmed.ncbi.nlm.nih.gov/31992387 Retrieved March 2021.

> Prove me wrong. Provide me with the record, which demonstrates how the COVID-19 virus was purified. My FOI appeal is that it would be reasonable to any layperson and to any Judge that the NVRL should be able to prove the existence of the COVID-19 virus and the only way to do this is to purify it.
>
> Please let me know by what date I can expect a decision on the FOI review.

On 22 June 2020, I received the following response to my appeal from Julian Bostridge, Director of Legal Services at University College Dublin.

> **Reference: FOI12_1_544 Internal Review**
>
> Dear Mr McCumiskey,
>
> In the original decision, Ms Scanlan refused part 1 of your request on grounds that the University do not hold records to answer your request (Section 15 (1) (a)).
>
> I have now conducted an internal review in accordance with Section 21 of the Act. I wish to inform you that I affirm the original decision.
>
> The University's position is that matters of academic debate cannot be conducted under FOI and we would not regard academic research material as administrative records of an FOI body that would make them available for release under the legislation. The NVRL have advised that they do not culture live SARS-CoV-2 or purify SARS CoV 2 antigens. They detect SARS-CoV-2 RNA in diagnostic samples, as per the PCR assay that was shared with you previously. As such, there are no relevant records held and no further searches that may be taken for records that

would provide an answer to your query. Section 15 (1) (a) of the FOI applies.

The University is committed to its obligations under the Act to provide requesters with access to records held by it and with reasons for its decisions that affect them. In this case, we regret that we cannot assist you further.

Given the gravity of the situation with the Lockdown, the next day, I appealed this internal review to the Office of the Information Commissioner.

Proving the Existence of Pathogenic Viruses

My position is that pathogenic viruses do not exist. There is no proof that any alleged pathogenic virus exists, such as the latest corona virus, which caused the Lockdown: COVID-19 / 2019-nCoV / SARS-CoV-2. This virus has multiple names in common usage; I believe SARS-CoV-2 (**S**evere **A**cute **R**espiratory **S**yndrome—**Co**rona **V**irus-**2**) is the most current name for this alleged pathogenic virus.

There is also no proof that the mumps virus, the measles virus, the rubella virus, HIV virus, bird flu virus H5N1, swine flu virus H1N1 nor indeed any other allegedly pathogenic virus exists.

If any of these allegedly pathogenic viruses existed, it would be possible to purify them.

It is possible to purify so-called bacteriophages, which have a diameter ranging from 100nm. A nanometre is one billionth of a metre or 1×10^{-9} m. Thousands of different types of bacteriophages have been purified using the density gradient centrifugation technique.

The NVRL have correctly stated to me in multiple FOI requests that "No Record Exists" in relation to the purification of any alleged pathogenic virus such as the measles virus and the SARS-CoV-2 virus. They are absolutely correct in stating that no scientist has ever purified any alleged pathogenic virus.

The scientists have been unable to purify any alleged pathogenic virus because they do not exist.

The entire country was quarantined because of the alleged existence of the SARS-CoV-2 virus. The Lockdown has caused considerable economic hardship. Therefore, I think it is reasonable to expect UCD NVRL to be able to provide proof, i.e. to provide the record, which definitively proves that the SARS-CoV-2 virus exists.

In order to prove the existence of a pathogenic virus one would have to purify it, photograph it, measure its diameter, and biochemically characterise its nucleic acid and the protein shell surrounding it.

FOI Request to UCD and the use of "record" for FOI purposes

I understand that under the FOI Act, UCD NVRL "is responsible for considering only those records that it holds or that are under its control" (Stephen Rafferty, Case Number 160377, 17 January 2017).

My latest FOI request to UCD NVRL was for two separate records:

> *1) I am looking for a scientific paper, which demonstrates how the Novel Coronavirus was purified? Surely, if the NVRL is able to detect the Novel Coronavirus, it should also be able to demonstrate how it is purified?*
>
> *2) I am also requesting how the NVRL would currently detect the Novel Coronavirus? Do you detect RNA*

(RiboNucleic Acid) in patients with pneumonia and then assume that the presence of RNA is equivalent to the presence of the Novel Coronavirus? Or do you use other indirect means for detecting the Novel Coronavirus?"

1. UCD NVRL correctly replied that the first record does not exist—i.e. no scientist has ever purified the Novel Coronavirus. I know that this is correct because the Novel Coronavirus does not exist, nor indeed does any other alleged pathogenic virus.

2. UCD NVRL provided me with the second record "Detection of 2019 novel coronavirus (2019-nCoV) by real-time RT-PCR". I would like to point out to the OIC that UCD NVRL explicitly did not create this record; rather the record is used by UCD NVRL to detect the Novel Coronavirus (2019-nCoV).

   The "Background" section of this detection methodology, in the very first sentence, states the truth: "as virus isolates are unavailable". The Aim of the paper also states the truth: "We aimed to develop and deploy robust diagnostic methodology for use in public health laboratory settings without having virus material available."

3. This scientific paper for detecting the Novel Coronavirus (SARS-CoV-2) explicitly states that the virus itself was not purified: "without having virus material available". The technique used is to detect RNA strands using real-time RT-PCR, which they believe are similar to the RNA strands from the original SARS virus (SARS-CoV-1). However, this belief is based on an illusion, because they have also never purified the SARS-CoV-1 virus.

4. In summary, UCD NVRL are correct in stating that "NO Record Exists" in relation to the purification of the

SARS CoV-2 virus, the measles virus etc. The reason why "No Record Exists" is because these allegedly pathogenic viruses do not exist.

5. What I want is for UCD NVRL to elaborate on why "No Record Exists" and why they continue to believe in the existence of these allegedly pathogenic viruses, despite the incontrovertible fact that it is impossible to purify them.

Queries for UCD NVRL

1. I want UCD NVRL to state the possible ranges of the estimated diameters of the measles virus and the SARS-CoV-2 virus, as two examples of allegedly pathogenic viruses.
2. UCD NVRL told an OIC investigator, Stephen Rafferty, in his report (Case Number 160377) dated 17 January 2017, that the density gradient centrifugation technique was "an old method" which had been "superseded by more modern techniques".
3. Can UCD NVRL state what technique(s) is/are currently used to purify any alleged pathogenic virus? May I be presented with the paper where a scientist has purified the measles virus and the SARS-CoV-2 virus using these "more modern techniques"?
4. I want UCD NVRL to explain why it is not possible to purify the SARS-CoV-2 virus nor the measles virus.
5. I want UCD NVRL to explain why it is not possible to purify the SARS-CoV-2 virus nor the measles virus using the density gradient centrifugation technique. This query is particularly relevant because this technique has been successfully used to purify thousands of different types of bacteriophages, with a similar diameter to all alleged pathogenic viruses.

I received the following prompt response from the investigator, Stephen Rafferty of the Office of the Information Commissioner on July 20 2020.

Our Reference: OIC-92955-C5Y6Z6

Your Reference: FOI12_1_544

Mr James McCumiskey

Re: Application for review under the Freedom of Information Act 2014 (the FOI Act)

Dear Mr McCumiskey

I refer to your the application for review by the Information Commissioner of the decision of the University College Dublin (UCD) where you submitted a two-part request seeking records *"1) for a scientific paper, which demonstrates how the Novel Coronavirus was purified? Surely, if the NVRL is able to detect the Novel Coronavirus, it should also be able to demonstrate how it is purified? And 2) requesting how the NVRL would currently detect the Novel Coronavirus? Do you detect RNA (RiboNucleic Acid) in patients with pneumonia and then assume that the presence of RNA is equivalent to the presence of the Novel Coronavirus? Or do you use other indirect means for detecting the Novel Coronavirus?"*

I note that UCD in its original decision dated 22 May 2020, agreed to grant partial access to the second-part of your request by providing you with an article but refused in full under the first-part of the request under S15(1)(a) on the basis that the documents sought by you did not exist. You then sought an internal review of this decision on 1 June 2020, in relation to the first-part of the request and this was affirmed by UCD on 22 June 2020. You then applied to this Office on 23 June 2020, for a review of this decision. This case has been assigned to me for investigation and recommendation.

Request for submissions

At the outset, I sent a request for submissions to UCD asking them to address the refusal of your review under S15(1)(a) and invited them to respond as to the general terms as to why they believe such documents do not exist. I also asked them to respond to the specific queries that you sent to this Office in the form of submissions and also for them to provide any comments they wished to make.

Section 15(1)(a)

The FOI Act is about access to records that exist and an FOI Body is not required under this Act to create a record, where none exists, to address the questions that you have put forward. This Office generally takes the approach that requests for information under FOI are requests for records containing that information. In this regard, I note that UCD's position in both its original and internal review is that it does not hold records relating to your request. For the purposes of this review, UCD were asked to provide this Office with more detail as to how and why it does not hold records relevant to your original request. Such a response may, for example, refer to the type of techniques used by the National Virus Reference Laboratory (the NVRL) or any other relevant information in support of UCD's decision to refuse the applicant's request on the basis that it does not and would not hold relevant records. I have outlined for you the queries put to UCD below and would be grateful if you are responding if you could adopt the numbering previously used.

UCD's General Comments

UCD commented that it has previously responded to FOI requests from you (FOI/800; FOI/830; FOI/840; FOI/979, FOI/1154, FOI12_1_064) in which you have disputed the existence of various viruses and sought records of the National Virus Reference Laboratory (NVRL) in support of your views. On each occasion decision-makers found that the request could not be answered, and the request was refused under Section 15(1) (a) of the Act (or Section 10(1) (a)) in relation to requests processed under the preceding legislation). Internal reviews were carried out and affirmed for FOI/800, FOI840, FOI979 and FOI1154. The decisions of UCD for FOI/800, FOI/840 were appealed to the OIC but investigation was discontinued on each occasion. FOI/1154 was also appealed to the OIC, where the decision was affirmed. In this case under review, a file was opened for the case under reference FOI12_1_544 and an acknowledgement and decision were issued to you. UCD acknowledges that the decision did not issue within statutory timeframe.

General Queries put to UCD

1. If UCD's position is that the record(s) sought do not exist, please clarify whether it is their position that the record(s) a) never existed (e.g. were never created or received) OR b) may have existed at some stage, but do not currently exist.

2. If it is UCD's position that the record(s) never existed, please explain why this is the case (e.g. if the normal practices and procedures of their organisation would not lead to the creation or retention of such record(s), please explain this position in detail).

3. Where the record(s) no longer exist, please explain what has occurred and provide details (and a copy) of the relevant Record Retention Policy and destruction instruction/policy document, indicating clearly the sections which apply to the records at issue, if such documentation exists.

> *UCD responded to all three above queries (1-3) by stating that they can confirm that their position is that it does not hold and has never held, the records sought.* ***You have asked for record held by UCD that demonstrate how the Novel Coronavirus was purified. The NVRL have confirmed that they do not employ the methodologies referenced in the request and therefore do not hold records to provide an answer to the requestor.*** *The NVRL do not culture live SARS-CoV-2 or purify SARS-CoV-2 antigen. While records may exist in the public domain to answer the request, as the NVRL do not carry out these techniques, no records are held by UCD to answer the request.*

<u>Specific Queries from you that you wished UCD to address</u>

In your application to this Office, you provided a submission entitled "COVID-19 Virus—Proving the Existence of Pathogenic Viruses". In this submission, you outlined your position and stated that in multiple previous FOI requests that the NVRL are correct in stating that "No Record Exists" in relation to the purification of the SARS- CoV-2 virus, the measles virus etc. The reason why "No Record Exists" is because these allegedly pathogenic viruses do not exist. You then set out some queries that you wish UCD to address as follows in queries (4-8) below and their responses to these queries are indented below each question:-

4. What the applicant appears to seek is for the UCD NVRL to elaborate on is why "No Record Exists" and why it continues to believe in the existence of these allegedly pathogenic viruses, despite the incontrovertible fact that it is impossible to purify them.

> ***What the requestor is looking for are matters of academic debate and we believe that such matters cannot be debated under FOI.*** *However, as stated above UCD do not hold records to answer the request, as the NVRL do not employ the methodologies referenced.*

5. Can UCD NVRL state the possible ranges of the estimated diameters of the measles virus and the SARS-CoV-2 virus, as two examples of allegedly pathogenic viruses.

> *As per previous requests from the requestor, UCD interprets questions, or requests for information as a request for records held by them and is not required to create a record to answer a request. The NVRL do not employ the methodologies reference, however there are significant peer reviewed publications and information available at the WHO website. Please see attached references which may address some of the questions posed by the requestor, as follows: a) JKMS: Virus Isolation from the First Patient with SARS-CoV-2 in Korea b) Isolation and rapid sharing of the 2019 novel coronavirus (SARS-CoV-2) from the first patient diagnosed with COVID-19 in Australia c) Nature Communications: Promotion of virus assembly and organization by the measles virus matrix protein d) Bulletin of the Osaka Medical College: Analysis of Morphology and Infectivity of Measles Virus Particles*

6. In a previous FOI request to this Office, UCD NVRL told this Office (Case Number 160377), that the density gradient centrifugation technique was "an old method" which had been "superseded by more modern

techniques". What technique(s) is/are currently used to purify any alleged pathogenic virus? He wishes to be presented with the paper where a scientist has purified the measles virus and the SARS-CoV-2 virus using these "more modern techniques"?

As outlined above the NVRL do not purify pathogenic viruses, thus they hold no records to show how those techniques are used. *The NVRL have provided the following explanation to further explain why they do not hold the requested records: "Traditional diagnostic virological techniques were based upon isolating the virus in tissue culture and further characterising the virus by specific immunofluorescent antibodies which are directed against specific viral proteins. Alternatively, a specific well characterised antibody could be mixed with the virus isolated in the tissue culture. This mixture is then added to a cell line and if the antibody is specific for the virus, there will be no replication in the cell line. This is called "in vitro" virus neutralisation and can characterise the virus. It is therefore not necessary to purify the virus to classify the virus."*

7. The applicant wants UCD NVRL to explain why it is not possible to purify the SARS-CoV-2 virus nor the measles virus.

> As per previous requests from the requestor, UCD interprets questions, or requests for information as a request for records held by them and is not required to create a record to answer a request. **The NVRL has no requirement to purify SARS-CoV-2 or measles virus and although there are methods in the public domain which describe such techniques, UCD do not hold such records.** They suggest that it would be more beneficial if vaccine manufacturers were contacted by the applicant, as they would be in a better position to discuss purification of viruses.

8. Please explain why it is not possible to purify the SARS-CoV-2 virus nor the measles virus using the density gradient centrifugation technique. This query is particularly relevant because this technique has been successfully used to purify thousands of different types of bacteriophages, with a similar diameter to all alleged pathogenic viruses.

> *As per previous requests from the requestor, UCD interprets questions, or requests for information as a request for records held by them and is not required to create a record to answer a request.* ***The NVRL has no requirement to purify SARS-CoV-2 or measles virus, although there are methods in the public domain which describe such techniques. However, as discussed in previous correspondence, density gradient centrifugation is a method which is not commonly used today and is not a method used by the NVRL.*** *They suggest that it would be beneficial if vaccine manufacturers were contacted by the applicant as they would be in a better position to discuss purification of viruses.*

Conclusion and Next Steps

The purpose of this letter is to inform you of the steps taken by UCD to show that all reasonable steps appear to have been taken to establish the whereabouts if any of the records sought insofar as they are held by and within their control. They also state again that no records exist in relation to the records in question. I am presently of the view that UCD have been correct in their application of Section 15(1)(a) of the FOI Act as it applies here and you may now wish to consider withdrawing your application for review at this time as there appears to be nothing further for this Office to review on the basis that there are no records in existence as you yourself are also of this view.

I was very happy with the Office of the Information Commissioner and the investigator Stephen Rafferty. He put my queries to the NVRL and although they did not seriously address them, their responses are revealing. The most significant admission by the NVRL was that they do not purify any viruses and in particular, they have not purified the SARS-CoV-2 virus. I was and am still firmly of the opinion that their written admissions would be useful in a future legal case.

RT-PCR Test

With the introduction of the PCR test for SARS-CoV-2, we had a 'testdemic', an epidemic of testing, resulting in a 'casedemic', an epidemic of cases. We had an epidemic of positive test results, an epidemic of people who tested positive but did not have the severe symptoms of COVID such as SARS—Severe Acute Respiratory Syndrome. Most people who tested positive were not hospitalised; they self-isolated at home. Many people who tested positive, probably also had a flu and other alleged associated symptoms such as sensory losses of smell and taste but had no breathing difficulties; they all believed they had COVID because they tested positive and had some of the lesser associated symptoms.

PCR or Polymerase Chain Reaction is a DNA manufacturing technique invented by Kary Mullis, who received the Nobel Prize for chemistry in 1993. The virologists believe that the coronavirus has an RNA nucleus surrounded by a protein shell. The RNA is converted to DNA prior to it being multiplied by PCR. The process of converting RNA to DNA is called Reverse Transcription—RT. Once the RNA is converted to DNA it is then multiplied using PCR.

> Starting with one DNA strand, the strand is cleaved (split in two) and then complementary strands are allowed to grow, the same process that occurs in a cell during mitosis (cell division). So far, not so impressive, but through the magic of doubling, if this process is repeated 10 times you will have about 1,000 identical strands of DNA (Crowe, 2020:1).

Each round of doubling is called a cycle. Theoretically, the PCR cycle number at which DNA is detectable tells us the relative quantity of RNA at the onset. In simple terms, the more RNA available at the outset, the lower the cycle number required to detect it.

In an audio interview with David Crowe from *The Infectious Myth,* RT-PCR expert Professor Stephen Bustin stated that the number of cycles should be limited to a maximum of 35 (Crowe, 2020:2). 35 cycles means a multiplication of the original sample by over 34 billion.

Professor Drosten's test had 45 cycles to determine whether someone tested positive for COVID. What that means is that the higher the cycle count on a PCR test, the more people will test positive. The cycle count of 45 is considerably higher than the recommended 35 by Professor Stephen Bustin. 45 cycles means a multiplication of the original sample by over 35 trillion. Thus, 45 cycles is over 1,000 times bigger than 35 cycles.

Other authors claim that the cycle count should not exceed 30: "But, an analytical result with a Ct value of 45 is scientifically and diagnostically absolutely meaningless (a reasonable Ct-value should not exceed 30)" (Borger, 2020).

The way to end the casedemic is simple: lower the number of cycles, and you automatically significantly lower the number of positive test results.

PCR tests for a virus is the definitive proof that virology is not a science but instead is wirrology! PCR tests for the coronavirus are 'wirr' or complete nonsense. How can you detect a virus using PCR, when you have never purified the virus in the first place and determined its genome?

What exactly are you multiplying using PCR? It transpires that you are multiplying bits of RNA, which are believed to belong to a coronavirus. However, these fragments of RNA can also exist in a papaya fruit.[24] Thus, PCR tests for the coronavirus (or indeed any virus) are completely meaningless.

I am not in any way criticising the PCR technology itself: I am merely criticising its use for the detection of the SARS-CoV-2 virus or indeed any other alleged virus.

The following extract is from Professor Christian Drosten's paper: Detection of 2019 novel coronavirus (2019-nCoV) by real-time RT-PCR (Drosten, 2020).

> **Aim:** We aimed to develop and deploy robust diagnostic methodology for use in public health laboratory settings without having virus material available.

---

24 https://iceagenow.info/papaya-yes-the-fruit-tests-positive-for-the-virus/ Retrieved March 2021

> **Methods:** Here we present a validated diagnostic workflow for 2019-nCoV, its design relying on close genetic relatedness of 2019-nCoV with SARS coronavirus, making use of synthetic nucleic acid technology.
>
> **Results:** The workflow reliably detects 2019-nCoV, and further discriminates 2019-nCoV from SARS-CoV.

Professor Drosten expressly admits there is no virus material available. The reality is that nobody has ever purified the SARS-CoV-2 virus. He is relying on the close genetic characteristics of SARS-CoV-2 to the SARS coronavirus. The PCR test is testing for short genetic sequences, which are ascribed to the SARS coronavirus. Again, nobody has ever purified the original SARS coronavirus. Professor Drosten claims to be able to differentiate between two viruses, which have never been purified in the first place.

If the SARS-CoV-2 virus existed, it would be possible to accurately determine its genome sequence and to then design and develop a PCR test to detect it. One cannot use a PCR test to detect something that does not exist.

The Orchestration of the Corona Crisis[25]

January 1 2020 Professor Christian Drosten from Charité in Berlin claims to have developed a PCR test, with which one can reliably prove the presence of the new corona virus.

25 The first two dates and information came from: Dr Stefan Lanka, 2020:2. The next dates and information came from: Professor Michel Chossudovsky, 2021.

January 21 2020 The WHO recommended his testing process to China and all nations as a reliable test process.

January 21-24, 2020 The annual meeting of the World Economic Forum (WEF) in Davos discussed an initiative for a COVID vaccine.

January 30 2020 The WHO confirmed that there were 83 positive cases outside China, including 5 in the US, 3 in Canada, 4 in France and 4 in Germany. WHO launched a Public Health Emergency of International Concern (PHEIC) based on these exceptionally low numbers.

January 31 2020 President Trump suspended air travel with China based on 5 cases of SARS in the USA.

February 20 2020 the WHO Director General Tedros held a press conference warning that a pandemic was imminent: "I believe the window of opportunity is still there, but that the window is narrowing." The confirmed cases outside China were then 1,073. When you relate this number to the world population, it is statistically irrelevant.

March 11, 2020 The WHO Director General officially declared a worldwide pandemic. At this time, the number of confirmed cases outside China was of the order of 44,279 with 1,440 deaths. Although these numbers are much higher, they are still not statistically relevant. Nonetheless, the United Nations instructed its 193 member states to implement the lockdown in order to help resolve the worldwide pandemic.

In contrast, tuberculosis is according to the WHO, the world's most dangerous infectious disease. Approximately 10 million people are diagnosed with tuberculosis every year and about 4,000 people die every day. Around 1.5 million people died in 2018 from tuberculosis.[26]

Tuberculosis is a disease associated with poverty and contrary to what the WHO says it is not contagious. However, the numbers of people dying from tuberculosis on a daily basis are significantly higher than those that are allegedly dying from COVID-19. The comparison between COVID-19 and tuberculosis proves that the Corona Crisis was orchestrated.

Compulsory Mask Wearing

Before COVID, the most important group of people who regularly wore facemasks were surgical teams working in an operating theatre. The rationale behind them wearing surgical facemasks is to prevent postoperative wound infections. The rationale is to prevent the surgical team from infecting the patient.

In 1991, a study was published in Sweden, which measured the incidence of postoperative wound infections with and without the use of surgical facemasks. 3,088 patients were included in the study over a period of 115 weeks. 1,537 operations were performed with facemasks, 73 wound infections were recorded, which is an incidence of 4.7%. 1,551 operations were performed without facemasks, 55 wound infections were recorded, which is an incidence of 3.5%. The difference between the respective percentages was not statistically significant. Masks "have not been

26 https://www.dw.com/en/who-tuberculosis-is-the-worlds-deadliest-infectious-disease/a-52895167 Retrieved September 2021

proven to protect the patient operated by a healthy operating team". Their recommendation: "These results indicated that the use of face masks might be reconsidered" (Tunevall, 1991).

The important point to note in this 1991 study is that despite the fact that there was no reduction in postoperative wound infections, worldwide, surgical teams continued to wear facemasks. This demonstrates the power of the Biomedical Paradigm. Despite the fact that there is no evidence supporting the wearing of facemasks, the surgical teams continue to wear them. The belief that they may 'spread germs' is much stronger than the actual scientific evidence.

Mask wearing became compulsory in the COVID era. FFP stands for **F**iltering **F**ace **P**iece. It is a half facemask covering the mouth and nose. FFP masks are dust masks to protect the wearer against inhaling airborne particulates. FFP1 masks filter 80% of dust particles; FFP2 masks filter 94% of dust particles and FFP3 masks filter 99% of dust particles. FFP1 masks filter dust particles greater than 5,000nn; FFP2 masks filter dust particles between 2,000 – 5,000nm and FFP3 masks filter dust particles around 2,000nm.[27]

If we assume that the SARS-CoV-2 virus is a giant virus with a diameter of 200nm, then how could any facemask filter away such a small particle? Even if viruses existed, high quality facemasks would not be able to offer any protection. Even within the confines of the Biomedical

27 http://www.dustmasksdirect.co.uk/different-types-of-dust-mask Retrieved March 2021

Paradigm, there is no justification for wearing facemasks given the size of the alleged viruses.

There is another agenda behind wearing facemasks and I think it one of subjugation, instilling fear into people so that they will be eager to be vaccinated against a phantom virus.

Gaslighting[28]

We are undergoing the world's largest ever gaslighting operation where we are being persuaded by very elaborate means that there is a pandemic, that we must wear facemasks to protect ourselves from the SARS-CoV-2 virus, that we must practice social distancing and that we should in effect quarantine ourselves from other people including our relatives and friends. The gaslighting is so effective that the vast majority of us wear facemasks without complaint and some even feel that they have the right and obligation to castigate the few people that refuse to wear them.

The COVID-19 gaslighting operation has been remarkably successful, so much so, that most people are now eager to be vaccinated.

Manifestly Unreasonable Requests

28 To 'gaslight' someone is to make him or her constantly doubt themselves, their actions and their perception of reality. The COVID-19 gaslighting operation makes its victims doubt their perception of reality and convinces them that there is a pandemic, despite empirical evidence to the contrary.

I emailed the National Virus Reference Laboratory on Thursday 7 January 2021 out of mischief really, asking them for the diameter of viruses. I had already asked this question previously, and they had responded with their customary 'No Record Exists'. I expected them to reply that they had previously answered my FOI request, which they had.

However, the response from Debbie Scanlan, Information Compliance Manager, on Friday 26 February 2021 surprised me, because she wrote that my repeated FOI requests were "manifestly unreasonable".

> Reference: FOI12_1_673
>
> Dear Mr McCumiskey,
>
> I refer to your request under the Freedom of Information Act 2014, for access to records held by the University.
>
> You requested, "I request from the NVRL at UCD the diameter of the following viruses in nm (nanometers) Mumps, Measles, Rubella, SARS-CoV-2, SARS-COV-1."
>
> The FOI Act provides for a right of access to records held by FOI bodies. The Act does not require FOI bodies to answer questions or to create records, which do not exist. Where a request is made in the form of a question or for specific information, it will be treated as a request for relevant records that exist as of the date of the request that contain the information sought.
>
> Having considered the provisions of the Act, I must refuse access to the requested records as they do not exist. As per our previous decisions in response to requests of a similar nature received from you, the NVRL have advised that they do not isolate pathogenic viruses and therefore

they do not hold records relating to the diameter of such viruses. The NVRL have the technical ability to detect pathogenic viruses.

As an FOI body, we are committed to giving assistance, where possible, to a person who is seeking access to records under the Act. As advised the requested records do not exist, however I have been advised by the NVRL that the following website may assist you with your query: https://www.rki.de/EN/Content/infections/Diagnostics/NatRefCentresConsultantLab/CONSULAB/VirusExplorer.html

As no relevant records held and no further searches that may be taken for records that would provide an answer to your query, I must apply section 15(1) of the Act, which states; 15. (1) A head to whom an FOI request is made may refuse to grant the request where—(a) the record concerned does not exist or cannot be found after all reasonable steps to ascertain its whereabouts have been taken.

In arriving at my decision to refuse your request, I have also considered the exemption provided for in section 15(1)(g) of the FOI Act.

Over the past number of years, my office has dealt with numerous requests from you, relating to the detection and isolation of various pathogenic viruses. Your requests for records were refused as no records were held by the university to answer your requests. When you appealed a decision either to my office and/or to the Office of the Commissioner, the original decision has been upheld in each case. The matters raised is your requests refer to academic research, rather than the administration records of the University and cannot be dealt with under the Freedom of Information Act.

> Having considered the pattern of your repeated requests directed to the University and elsewhere, I find that they must be regarded as manifestly unreasonable, within the terms of S.15(1)(g) of the FOI Act, which states;
>
> > 15. (1) A head to whom an FOI request is made may refuse to grant the request where—the request is, in the opinion of the head, frivolous or vexatious or forms part of a pattern of manifestly unreasonable requests from the same requester or from different requesters who, in the opinion of the head, appear to have made the requests acting in concert.

The link they provided me is to "VirusExplorer DEM", a database maintained by the Robert Koch Institute, which provides electron microscopy images of 'viruses'; They are committing scientific fraud because they are misrepresenting these images to be those of purified viruses.

On Sunday 7 March 2021, after much reflection, I made my final FOI appeal to University College Dublin. My prayer was that the Director of Legal Service might for once investigate my claims and not reply with a perfunctory and vacuous 'No Record Exists'.

> Dear Mr Julian Bostridge, Director of Legal Services at UCD,
>
> I am appealing another "No Record Exists" FOI response from Debbie Scanlan, Information Compliance Manager at UCD Freedom of Information Unit.
>
> To reiterate my long-held position: Pathogenic viruses do not exist. The SARS-CoV-2 virus does not exist, neither does the mumps, measles, rubella, HIV, H1N1 viruses etc.

The latest FOI response from the National Virus Reference Laboratory (NVRL) proves my point: ".. the NVRL have advised that they do not isolate pathogenic viruses and therefore do not hold records relating to the diameter of such viruses".

I accept the fact that the NVRL and University College Dublin can under FOI hide behind the legalities of the fact that "No Record Exists". I am stating emphatically that no record exists because pathogenic viruses do not exist. UCD NVRL obfuscate the issue by saying that: "The matters raised in your requests refer to academic research, rather than the administration records of the University and cannot be dealt with under the Freedom of Information Act". I found it ironic and amusing that you regard my "repeated requests" as "manifestly unreasonable". Really! I feel the same way about your repeated "No Record Exists".

However, my FOI requests go way beyond FOI and now question the standing of UCD as a scientific institution and reputable university. If you bother to question your colleagues in the School of Biology and Environmental Sciences, you will discover that they unlike their NVRL colleagues, they use Density Gradient Centrifugation to purify bacteriophages. The diameter of bacteriophages ranges from 24nm to 200nm. Bacteriophages do exist, they have been purified, photographed, their dimensions measured and have been biochemically characterised both the nucleus and protein shell. All alleged pathogenic viruses range in diameter from 5nm to 300nm. The measles virus for example is alleged to be pleiomorphic (irregularly shaped) with a diameter between 120nm-250nm. I understand that corona viruses are alleged to have a diameter between 80nm-120nm. My point is reasonable and logical: if it is possible to purify bacteriophages, which are of a similar size to all alleged viruses, then why is it not possible to purify pathogenic viruses?

Three years ago I suggested a control experiment to your NVRL colleagues: Purify a bacteriophage using density gradient centrifugation and as a control experiment attempt to purify a pathogenic virus (mumps, measles or even SARS-CoV-2) from a blood sample / sputum sample / swab sample. This simple control experiment would take a few hours to perform and would provide proof that these alleged pathogenic viruses do not exist.

If the UCD School of Biology are unwilling to carry out this simple and inexpensive experiment, then UCD forfeits its right to be classed as a university, dedicated to the pursuit of scientific truth. In fact UCD is engaged in scientific misconduct of the utmost gravity, because the scientists are unwilling to query their underlying assumptions that the Germ Theory of Disease is correct and that pathogenic viruses exist.

This scientific misconduct has now become a criminal fraud because UCD is making a false representation of fact—claiming that viruses exist, when they know that it is impossible to purify them—and that there must be genuine "academic debate" as to whether they exist or not. UCD NVRL have made this false representation to the Irish government, who have instituted the must draconian lockdown measures against a fictitious virus—SARS-CoV-2. In fact, it goes way beyond scientific fraud and into the realm of crimes against humanity.

I know that "No Record Exists" in relation to the purification of viruses because they do not exist. Prove me wrong. Create the record: attempt to purify any alleged

> pathogenic virus and write up the results. I do not fear scientific truth. Do you?

Mr Julian Bostridge, Director of Legal Services replied to me on Wednesday 21 April 2021. While polite, he 'doubled-down' on my "manifestly unreasonable requests".

> The FOI Act provides for a right of access to records held by FOI bodies. The Act does not require FOI bodies to answer questions or to create records to answer a request. The NVRL have confirmed on repeated occasions, that they do not isolate pathogenic viruses, have no requirement to do so and therefore they do not hold records relating to the diameter of such viruses. Your internal review request, dated 07/03/21 appears to accept this position, stating, "I accept the fact that the NVRL and University College Dublin can under FOI hide behind the legalities of the fact that "No Record Exists". I am stating emphatically that no record exists because pathogenic viruses do not exist."
>
> The other points of you appeal relate to matters of academic debate, which cannot be conducted under FOI. You requested that in order to answer your request, the University create a new record as follows, "I know that "No Record Exists" in relation to the purification of viruses because they do not exist. Prove me wrong. Create the record: attempt to purify any alleged pathogenic virus and write up the results. I do not fear scientific truth. Do you?". As advised, the FOI Act does not require the university to answer questions or create records which do not exist, and I find Ms Scanlan correctly relied on section 15 (1) (a) to refuse your request.
>
> I have also considered Ms Scanlan's application of section 15 (1)(g) for the FOI Act, which states:

> 15. (1) A head to whom an FOI request is made may refuse to grant the request where— g) the request is, in the opinion of the head, frivolous or vexatious or forms part of a pattern of manifestly unreasonable requests from the same requester or from different requesters who, in the opinion of the head, appear to have made the requests acting in concert.

> I have reviewed your previous FOI requests and internal review requests for records relating to pathogenic viruses over the past number of years and find that the decision makers and internal reviewers reached the same decision each time, in that the records you seek do not exist. Subsequent external reviews to the Office of the Information Commissioner were either discontinued or the decision of the University upheld. I find therefore, that your repeated requests for information of a similar nature, that you yourself have said you know not to exist, do form a pattern of manifestly unreasonable requests and that Ms Scanlan was correct in relying on section 15(1)(g) to refuse your request.

I understand the power of belief systems. I understand the enormous hold the Germ Theory of Disease has over the vast majority of humanity. Despite that, I do not understand why when facts are formulated in a clear and unambiguous manner, that the scientists cannot question and test them. The vacuous response from the scientists at the National Virus Reference Laboratory in Dublin has been very disappointing over a prolonged period.

The responses of the FOI officers and the Director of Legal Services were also disappointing. They are in effect backing the scientists at the NVRL. They are being minimalist in their interpretation of FOI legislation. No Record

Exists—that is it. They are not asking the obvious questions. Why is there no record? Why is it impossible to purify any pathogenic virus? What does the NVRL use of the phrase "academic debate" mean? Could it be that there is no evidence supporting the existence of pathogenic viruses and this is a topic of discussion among virologists?

It will take a real intellectual struggle to overcome one's education / indoctrination at school, university as well as one's professional career, and that is not easy, I do understand that. Nonetheless, if the scientists are interested in the truth, the scientific truth, as far as it is known at this moment in time, then this is what must be done.

At some point in one's life, particularly as one gets older, what matters most: money and all the goods it can buy, career, prestige or personal honour and integrity, and that one is pursuing truth for the benefit of humanity? Truth is much more important than self-preservation and self-aggrandisement. We cannot change the truth to suit ourselves. We have to accommodate ourselves to the truth. If our beliefs are wrong, we have to change them to fit in with the truth. Truth is. We have to pursue the truth because only it sets us free.

An Appalling Vista[29]

It is indeed an appalling vista that the medical profession, the virologists, the scientists, the media, the government, every public health official, every institution in the land and every single politician are wrong about the existence of the SARS-CoV-2 virus. It is an appalling vista that we have had lockdowns to prevent the spread of a phantom virus. The entire Corona Crisis is an appalling vista with far-reaching consequences for humanity. It is such an appalling vista that "every sensible person in the land would say that it cannot be right" that the virologists, medical doctors, public health officials and politicians are all spectacularly wrong.

The appalling vista argument is very powerful. It is such a powerful argument, that most people almost immediately and even instinctively dismiss anyone questioning the

29 The Irish Republican Army (IRA) bombed two busy pubs in Birmingham in 1974, which killed 21 people and injured 182 others. Six innocent Irishmen were convicted of the atrocity in 1975. They became known as the Birmingham Six. Lord Justice Denning made the "appalling vista" judgment in 1980 when he denied an appeal by the Birmingham Six against their wrongful conviction. His reasoning was,"*If the six men win, it will mean that the police are guilty of perjury, that they are guilty of violence and threats, that the confessions were invented and improperly admitted in evidence and the convictions were erroneous... This is such an appalling vista that every sensible person in the land would say that it cannot be right that these actions should go any further*". The "appalling vista" judgment was so important that the Birmingham Six were incarcerated for another eleven years until their release and exoneration in 1991. They each got about £1m in compensation.

existence of viruses. Some people even feel so confident in their belief that they vilify a dissenter as a 'virus-denier' or a 'science-denier'.

The following examples from my correspondence with lawyers about the missing viruses illustrates the power of the appalling vista argument. Ryanair correctly sued the Irish government in 2020 about the draconian travel restrictions. I contacted the two lawyers concerned about the fact that there is no proof that the SARS-CoV-2 virus exists. They never responded. In addition, a few years ago, I contacted a number of Irish lawyers specialising in medical malpractice but again, nobody responded. I think the reason why is because they assume that the underlying science is correct, that viruses must exist, and therefore that anyone questioning their existence must be wrong. It would be such an appalling vista if viruses did not exist that they must exist.

However, we have to move beyond the appalling vista argument, put it to one side, and coldly and rationally examine the evidence. The simple fact of the matter is that no one has ever purified any alleged pathogenic virus. Any reasonable person would have to agree, that if it is possible to purify bacteriophages, which are of an equivalent size to all alleged pathogenic viruses, then the fact that it is not possible to purify any alleged pathogenic virus can only mean one thing: viruses do not exist and cannot exist.

Prosecuting the Virologists for Scientific Fraud

The virologists should be prosecuted for scientific fraud, at the very least, if not for crimes against humanity.

They commit scientific fraud when they claim that viruses such as SARS-CoV-2 exist. They know that it is not possible to purify any alleged pathogenic virus using the standard technique—Density Gradient Centrifugation—and that it is possible to purify bacteriophages, which have a similar size to all alleged pathogenic viruses.

Dr Stefan Lanka believes the virologists could also be prosecuted for employment fraud because they masquerade as scientists but operate in a completely unscientific manner. They do not carry out any control experiments; they do not question their underlying assumptions; they do not investigate why nobody has ever purified any alleged pathogenic virus (Lanka, 2020:3).

The following facts must be determined in order to convict the virologists of scientific fraud:

1. The virologists have given specific names to newly identified viruses such as SARS-COV-1, SARS-CoV-2, HIV, H1N1 and H5N1, which by virtue of having a name, implies that they have been purified. However, nobody has ever purified a pathogenic virus—neither measles, HIV nor SARS-CoV-2;

2. It is possible to purify so-called bionts[30] (phages and giant viruses) using density gradient centrifugation. These bionts have a similar size to all alleged viruses;

30 A biont is a discrete unit of living matter. There is no such thing as viruses or pathogenic viruses. Dr Lanka now calls phages and 'giant viruses' bionts, and no longer uses the word 'virus' because it is derived from the Latin for poison and implies that what is being called a virus is pathogenic.

3. The virologists have published information about the sizes of all alleged viruses. For example, the measles virus is alleged to have a diameter of 120nm-250nm. It would be possible to purify the measles virus or the SARS-CoV-2 virus using Density Gradient Centrifugation—if they existed;

4. The fast that the virologists use PCR to 'detect the SARS-CoV-2 virus' implies that they have never purified the virus in the first place, because they are using an indirect method, which assumes that the virus exists;

5. When all is said and done, the issue is solely about the purification of a virus. Please cite the scientific publication where a virus has been purified!

The Corona Reset

All vaccines are dangerous, some more so than others, but they are all dangerous. The only good vaccine is one that is never used.

It is too early to say how toxic the vaccines are against the phantom SARS-CoV-2 virus. At this stage, given the amount of expert mainstream opinion opposed to the 'warp speed'[31] of the vaccine roll out, one would have to be very wary about the safety of all the various vaccines against SARS-CoV-2. However, I want to emphasise again

31 Operation Warp Speed (OWS) was a public—private partnership initiated by the US government to facilitate and accelerate the development, manufacturing, and distribution of COVID-19 vaccines, therapeutics, and diagnostics.

that all vaccines are dangerous and there is nothing new about the inherent toxicity of vaccines.

What is incredibly worrying is the manner in which the vaccine is being foisted on us, so much so that we may have to have a COVID passport to prove that we have been vaccinated, before we are allowed to fly, and even go to shops, restaurants or concerts in our own country.

However, while I do not doubt that there is an underlying malevolent agenda behind the orchestrated Corona Crisis, in my opinion, the real conspiracy, the ultimate conspiracy, is our collective belief in the Biomedical Paradigm, the Germ Theory of Disease and the existence of pathogenic viruses.

The Corona Reset will be the undoing of our belief in the existence of pathogenic viruses. Once most people understand that viruses cannot exist, there will have to be a broader examination of the Germ Theory of Disease and in particular Cellular Pathology—the belief that all life and disease originates from a cell.

Once most people accept that both of these key dogmas of medicine and biology are wrong, Dr Ryke Geerd Hamer's Five Biological Laws can be verified and implemented. The general acceptance of the Five Biological Laws will mean that we are no longer 'treated' by a medical professional, rather we understand why we got a particular cancer or disease and come up with our own personal solutions to resolve the biological conflict which caused our illness. The patient is in charge, and has to resolve his underlying biological conflict, thereby allowing the body to heal itself. This is in stark contrast with the current allopathic model, where the patient is 'treated' by an omnipotent medical doctor using allopathic means such as drugs, radical surgery, chemotherapy or radiotherapy to 'alleviate' the symptoms rather than attempt to resolve the underlying cause.

The Corona Reset will be the realisation that about 95% of medicine and biology is scientifically and medically wrong. The fact that viruses cannot exist will have far-reaching societal consequences, which transcend medicine and biology.

There will also have to be profound changes in how we are governed. It is incredible, that to my knowledge, only three countries in the world did not implement the full lockdown—Sweden, Tanzania and Belarus. It seems that our politicians are captured by the Biomedical Paradigm and cannot think rationally. Even within the mainstream narrative, how can it be acceptable to lockdown the world for a virus, which had a recovery rate in 2020 of over 99.90%? It makes no sense unless there is an underlying malevolent agenda.

The mainstream media enjoy vilifying anyone who questions the prevailing wisdom as a 'denier' a 'science denier' or a 'conspiracy theorist'. They are not operating as a free press giving voice to divergent opinions.

The Germ Theory of Disease is False and Viruses Cannot Exist

Germs do not cause disease. Saying that bacteria are the cause of disease is like saying that flies cause a dung-heap. Yes, when a cow creates a dung-heap, flies appear almost immediately. Yes, when a patient has tuberculosis, Tb bacilli are present but they do not cause it; in fact, they are our symbionts, our 'little helpers', helping us to return to full health. Although bacteria do exist and are present and active when the patient has all the symptoms of the associated disease, they do not cause it.

The Germ Theory of Disease does not work for bacteria because you cannot cause the same disease by ingesting the bacteria that allegedly cause that disease into another person.[32] Contrary to received wisdom, so-called bacterial diseases such as tuberculosis are not contagious.

The Germ Theory of Disease fails for viruses because they do not exist. Virology has now crippled, if not destroyed a significant section of the world economy with the repeated lockdowns. The abject failure of virology, medicine and science needs to be urgently rectified otherwise they will succeed in severely injuring and or killing hundreds of millions of people with their vaccines for SARS-CoV-2 or another new phantom virus.

Christians are familiar with the words of forgiveness Jesus offered those who were crucifying him: "Forgive them Father for they know not what they are doing". Dr Stefan Lanka writes sardonically that this should be rephrased for the virologists: "Forgive them Father, because they cannot admit that what they have learned and practice is not true and even more is dangerous or even deadly" (Lanka, 2020:1).

Despite what has happened, we must forgive them, the doctors, the scientists, the virologists and the politicians and move on and learn from our repeated mistakes over

32 Koch's third postulate.

hundreds if not thousands of years. They too are victims of the prevailing belief in the Germ Theory of Disease. This belief was confirmed to them as an accepted scientific truth during their secondary and tertiary education. They implicitly assumed it was true, just like the vast majority of us. Before we castigate them, we must examine our own conscience first and accept that most of us implicitly assumed that viruses exist. We too were captured by our collective belief in the Germ Theory of Disease.

The simple but profound aphorism we must clearly understand and accept is that the Germ Theory of Disease is false and viruses do not exist.

Sources

Pieter **Borger,** Ulrike Kämmerer et al, 2020, *External peer review of the RTPCR test to detect SARS-CoV-2 reveals 10 major scientific flaws at the molecular and methodological level: consequence for false positive results.*
https://cormandrostenreview.com/report/
Retrieved April 2021.

Dr Gerhard **Buchwald** MD, 1995, *Vaccination: A Business Based on Fear*
Books on Demand.

Genevieve **Carberry**, 2011, *Warning of more cases of flu vaccine disorder*
https://www.irishtimes.com/news/warning-of-more-cases-of-flu-vaccine-disorder-1.603289
Retrieved February 2021.

Fritjof **Capra**, 1983, *The Turning Point, Science, Society and the Rising Culture*
Fontana Paperbacks.

Professor Michel **Chossudovsky**, 2021, The 2020-21 Worldwide Corona Crisis: Destroying Civil Society, Engineered Economic Depression, Global Coup d'État and the "Great Reset".
https://www.globalresearch.ca/the-2020-worldwide-corona-crisis-destroying-civil-society-engineered-economic-depression-global-coup-detat-and-the-great-reset/5730652
Retrieved September 2021.

David **Crowe**, 2020:1, *Corona Virus Panic*
http://theinfectiousmyth.com/book/CoronavirusPanic.pdf
Retrieved March 2021.

David **Crowe**, 2020:2, *The Infectious Myth Episode 251 April 14 2020: Stephen Bustin on Challenges with RT-PCR*
https://infectiousmyth.podbean.com/e/the-infectious-myth-stephen-bustin-on-challenges-with-rt-pcr/
Retrieved May 2021.

Victor Corman, Christian **Drosten** et al, 2020, *Detection of 2019 novel coronavirus (2019-nCoV) by real-time RT-PCR*
https://pubmed.ncbi.nlm.nih.gov/31992387
Retrieved April 2021.

Gerald L. **Geison**, 1995, *The Private Science of Louis Pasteur*
Princeton University Press, Princeton, New Jersey.

Martin **Geddes**, 2021, *The Total Reset of Everything*
https://www.martingeddes.com/the-total-reset-of-everything/
Retrieved April 2021.

Dr Ryke Geerd **Hamer**, 2004, second edition, *Krebs und alle sog. Krankheiten, Kurze Einführung in die Germanisch neue Medizin (Cancer and all so-called Diseases, a brief introduction to the German New Medicine)*
Amici-di-Dirk.

Dr Muiris **Houston** MD, 2011, *Concerns over swine flu vaccine should not deter us from getting seasonal shot,*
Irish Times

https://www.irishtimes.com/news/concerns-over-swine-flu-vaccine-should-not-deter-us-from-getting-seasonal-shot-1.612453
Retrieved February 2021.

Ethel Douglas **Hume**, *2006, Béchamp or Pasteur? A Lost Chapter in the History of Biology.*
www.Béchamp.org
Retrieved April 2021.

Dr Stefan **Lanka,** 1995, *HIV; Reality or Artefact?* Continuum.
https://www.virusmyth.com/aids/hiv/slartefact.htm
Retrieved April 2021.

Dr Stefan **Lanka,** 2015:1, Dismantling the Virus Theory, The "measles virus" as an example
Wissenschafftplus 6/2015
https://wissenschafftplus.de/uploads/article/Dismantling-the-Virus-Theory.pdf Retrieved May 2021.

Dr Stefan **Lanka,** 2015:2, Entwicklung von Medizin and Menschheit. Wie geht es weiter?
(Development of medicine and humanity. How does it proceed?)
Wissenschafftplus 6/2015

Dr Stefan **Lanka,** 2020:1, *The Virus Misconception Part 1*
Wissenschafftplus 1/2020
https://wissenschafftplus.de/uploads/article/wissenschafftplus-the-virus-misconception-part-1.pdf
Retrieved April 2021.

Dr Stefan **Lanka,** 2020:2, *The Virus Misconception Part 11*

Wissenschafftplus 2/2020
https://wissenschafftplus.de/uploads/article/wissenschafftplus-the-virus-misconception-part-2.pdf
Retrieved April 2021.

Dr Stefan **Lanka,** 2020:3, *The initiators of the Corona Crisis have been clearly identified, VIROLOGISTS who claim the existence of disease-causing viruses exist are committing scientific fraud and must be prosecuted.*
https://wissenschafftplus.de/uploads/article/The-Initiators-of-the-Corona-Crisis-Have-Been-Clearly-Identified.pdf
Wissenschafftplus 4/2020,
Retrieved September 2021.

Eleanora **McBean**, 1977, *Swine Flu Expose*
http://whale.to/a/mcbean2.html
Retrieved September 2021.

James **McCumiskey,** 2009, *The Ultimate Conspiracy, The Biomedical Paradigm*
Literally Publishing.

Dr David **McGrogan**, 2021, *The Failed Strategy of Lockdown Sceptics: We appealed to Reason, Not Emotion*
https://lockdownsceptics.org/moral-truth-and-the-failed-strategy-of-lockdown-sceptics/
Retrieved March 2021.

Thomas **McKeown**, 1979, *The Role of Medicine,*
Basil Blackwell Publisher Ltd.

Dr Hans Ulrich **Niemitz**, 2003, *The German New Medicine, a new Natural Science*
http://www.newmedicine.ca/science.php
Retrieved March 2021.

Dan **Olmstead,** 2005, *The age of Autism, The Amish Anomaly*
https://www.upi.com/Science_News/2005/04/19/The-Age-of-Autism-The-Amish-anomaly/95661113911795/
Retrieved September 2021.

RB **Pearson**, *2006, Pasteur: Plagiarist, Imposter – The Germ Theory Exploded*
www.Béchamp.org
Retrieved April 2021.

Dr Saeed A **Qureshi**, 2021, *COVID-19: "Virus Isolation". Does the Virus Exist?*
https://thenewabnormal513330780.wordpress.com/2021/01/07/covid-19-virus-isolation-does-the-virus-exist/
Retrieved September 2021.

Dr Rustum **Roy**, 2002, *Science and Whole Person Medicine: Enormous Potential in a New Relationship*
https://journals.sagepub.com/doi/10.1177/027046702236890
Retrieved March 2021.

Ian **Sample**, 2005, *From frozen Alaska to the lab: a virus 39,000 times more virulent than flu*
https://www.theguardian.com/society/2005/oct/06/health.medicineandhealth2

Retrieved April 2021.

Liam **Scheff**, 2015, *The media campaign for AIDS tests*
https://www.aim.org/special-report/the-media-campaign-for-hiv-tests/
Retrieved March 2021.

Richard E **Shope** MD, 1958, *The R.E.Dyer Lecture: Influenza, History, Epidemiology, and Speculation*
Public Health Rep. 1958 Feb; 73(2): 165–179
http://europepmc.org/article/PMC/1951634
Retrieved April 2021.

Ian **Sinclair,** 1994, Fifth Edition, *Vaccination, The "Hidden" Facts*

Ursula **Stoll** & Dr Stefan Lanka, 2020, *Corona Weiter ins Chaos oder Chance für ALLE*, (Corona, Further into Chaos or an opportunity for us all)
Praxis Neue Medizin Verlag.

Gunnar **Tunevall**, 1991, *Postoperative wound infections and surgical face masks: a controlled study*
https://pubmed.ncbi.nlm.nih.gov/1853618
Retrieved April 2021.

Veronika **Widmer**, 2004, Impfen eine Entscheidung die Eltern treffen, (Vaccination, a decision parents make)
First Edition, klein-klein-verlag.

Shin Jie **Yong,** 2020, *Spread of Spanish Flu Was Never Experimentally Confirmed*

https://medium.com/microbial-instincts/spread-of-spanish-flu-was-never-experimentally-confirmed-9f91b37c4dd8
Retrieved March 2021.

Biological Terrain vs The Germ Theory
http://thehealthadvantage.com
Retrieved March 2021.

Acknowledgment

Dr Lanka has provided humanity an invaluable service by revealing the truth about pathogenic viruses calmly and repeatedly, and the fact that the Germ Theory of Disease and Cellular Pathology are false.

I acknowledge the late Karl Krafeld for his work in instigating citizen enquiry in 2000 along with Dr Stefan Lanka. I took up the challenge in Ireland and the UK and confirmed for myself that no one has ever purified a virus. I learned much more about virology than I ever wanted to know! However, this learning has been necessary, because I now understand the power of belief systems. I understand the power of the Biomedical Paradigm. I understand why the virologists, scientists and doctors have found it impossible to give up their belief in the Germ Theory of Disease.

I thank my sister Clodagh McCumiskey who inspired me to write this book in order to explain as coherently, objectively and succinctly as possible the truth behind the belief in viruses and the Germ Theory of Disease.

Over the years, I forwarded countless of my FOI requests to my friend - the renowned Swiss German New Medicine therapist - Harald Baumann. His reply to one of my emails was: "Well done! Regular drops of water will eventually perforate even the hardest stone... it's only a question of time". Thank you Harald for your unflagging support and wisdom.

I gratefully acknowledge the late David Crowe for his tremendous work in exposing the fact that viruses cannot exist. Had he lived, he would have thoroughly enjoyed exposing many more viral myths, conducting more interviews and publishing his book.

I thank other citizen journalists who interviewed me about the 'missing viruses'; the late Maurice Herman (Morris108); the Brizer Show; Open Your Mind Radio; Mark Windows—Windows on the World and Jime Sayaka from Subversive Thinking. Independent citizen journalists will expose the missing viruses - not the mainstream media.

I have been querying the existence of viruses for over 15 years. It has been a lonely path. I am grateful to those with whom I exchanged emails over the years, ordinary citizens with no medical training, who like me came to understand that viruses are theoretical constructs with no basis in biological reality. I am particularly grateful to Ulrike Berger, Felicia Popescu, Susanne Brix, John Wantling, Anthony Oatley, Kevin Boyle, 'Northern Tracey', Shannon Rowan, Russell Batten, Paul Joyce and countless others who helped me keep my sanity in a world gone mad.

I thank Karl Winn for his review of the manuscript and his helpful insights and suggestions.

I thank Nicola Mackin for publishing the book.

Finally, I gratefully acknowledge the help and guidance I received from the greatest Muse of them all – The Holy Spirit.

The Great Awakening

The lockdowns have caused profoundly negative economic and social consequences. When the Corona Crisis is over, there will be a prolonged Greater Depression with persistently high unemployment in the developed world. Many small businesses will never reopen.

The emotional consequence have been devastating: Grandparents did not meet or hug their grandchildren for months for fear of catching the virus; suicides have increased and mental health has deteriorated. As human beings, we require social contact and interaction.

Government has severely curtailed our civil and religious liberties; it has criminalised people for being warm human beings because they visited friends and families; it has forced us to wear masks in public spaces. We can no longer travel abroad without having to endure severe quarantine measures. There is now a division in society between the vaccinated and the un-vaccinated.

However bad the consequences are in the developed world they are even worse in the developing world with chronic hunger and even famine in the near future.

Famine in the developing world and a Greater Depression in the developed world—all because of a phantom virus?

Decades before the Corona Crisis, Dr Stefan Lanka provided the technical scientific arguments as to why no alleged pathogenic virus exists. The relevant scientific authorities proved they were not proper scientists because they could not question their own assumptions. They could not conceive of the possibility that the Germ Theory of Disease could be wrong. They could not carry out the necessary control experiments to prove that there is no evidence supporting the existence of viruses. They have proved that they are not real scientists.

The Corona Crisis provides us with the scientific and emotional arguments for ensuring that this never happens again. The Great Awakening will involve the Total Reset of Everything[19]—medicine, banking, money, law, taxation, government, media, education…

The Great Awakening will include many new insights and understandings. A key realisation will be that the central dogma of the Biomedical Paradigm—The Germ Theory of Disease—is false; Germs do not cause disease and viruses do not exist. Once we understand that the Germ Theory of Disease is wrong, we can swiftly discard all the other dogmas of allopathic medicine.

Dr Ryke Geerd Hamer's Five Biological Laws should then be finally tested and implemented, which would be a highly positive outcome from the corona catastrophe.

The lockdowns, the vaccines and the unnecessary ensuing economic and social hardship provides plenty of motivation to transform the Corona Crisis into a Corona Reset, to transform a catastrophe into a positive paradigm shift, a reset of medicine. I believe the Corona Reset will be the most significant reset of the Great Awakening.

---

19 The Total Reset of Everything is an essay by Martin Geddes.